PART ONE

INTRODUCTION

To see a world in a grain of sand and heaven in a wild flower, hold infinity in the palm of your hand and eternity in an hour.

—William Blake

A lot of exercise books are written by skinny people who always have been skinny, who never had a problem with fat. This book is written by a genetically fat person.

This is a book about fat, and how to get rid of it through just 12 minutes of aerobic exercise a day. These 12 minutes per day will change your metabolism; more importantly, they will change your outlook on life, so that you will feel younger than you have in years.

In 1977, I went to Rome for a vacation. As I climbed a flight of stairs to see the sights of the city, I thought my end was near. The years of smoking and drinking and no exercise had taken their toll. I resolved that when I returned to California I would finally get healthy. My first step would be to give up smoking my normal three packs of cigarettes a day.

I had always thought smoking was chic and sexy. And since I tend to be fat, whenever I tried to give up smoking I gained a lot of weight.

This time was no exception: I promptly put on 50 pounds. It was becoming difficult for me to get in and out of the new Corvette I had bought as an incentive to quit smoking. (I had made a bargain with myself: If I smoked I had to sell the Corvette; that was unthinkable.)

At about the same time, I was making regular visits to my doctor for chronic stomach trouble. He prescribed antacids and a new drug, Cimetidine, trade name Tagamet. Nothing seemed to work.

What bothered me the most about this experience with my doctor was that he could not find out what was wrong with me. He suggested that many people my age, 43, had chronic health problems, and that perhaps I should try to get used to being sick—and act my age. This infuriated me so much that I went to UCLA and bought every textbook on health, exercise, and nutrition I could find, and proceeded to read them all. I realized then that my health was in my own hands, and that it was up to me to learn how to keep myself healthy. Deciding to quit smoking was the first step. Now I was going to cure my stomach ailment and get rid of the 50 pounds.

One day, I ran into a Hollywood agent and an out-of-work actor who suggested that I come with them to a health club in Los Angeles. They took me to an advanced aerobics class. (Aerobic exercise is any exercise done fast enough to raise your heartbeat to its training level—certain exercises being better suited to this than others.[1]) Twenty minutes into the hour class, I could barely crawl on all fours as I tried to leave. I resolved to keep coming back, though, and over a period of six months

I gradually improved until I was doing the entire one-hour class.

As I got thinner (I lost 50 pounds), and began to enjoy the youthful feeling of movement, everything in my life improved. The increased oxygen intake caused by aerobics quickened my thought processes. The now well-known effects of endorphins released by strenuous exercise elevated and stabilized my emotions.[2] All the stomach problems I had been experiencing went away, never to return.

I was hooked. I not only gave up smoking, but all drugs—including alcohol and aspirin. Now, at 51, I am totally drug free, and have never felt better nor been more physically fit or productive in my life.

I should point out that my friends and I were almost always the only men in our class. Men either think the classes are "sissy" and wouldn't dream of wrecking their image by showing up at one or they have actually gone to a class, realized very quickly how physically demanding it is, and have snuck out the back door, panting, to remark to their friends from the racquetball court that it was a waste of time.

There is no question that women who regularly work out in good aerobics classes are in better shape than the men pumping iron and running the track on the other side of the club.

A good aerobics class is not so easy to find, though. Most health clubs offer little or no instruction. Their self-interest lies in your never returning after paying your initial fee. Many clubs I went to had no beginner class at all, and they held their aerobics class on a rug-covered concrete floor. Most of the regulars got severe shin splints from running on the concrete.

The impression one gets from these clubs is that you need to take the entire one-hour class to do yourself any good at all. As it turns out, after 12 minutes of strenuous aerobics, the next 12 minutes supply you with continually diminishing return for your effort. Furthermore, the second 12 minutes can cause damage to your body as you tire and are more prone to injury.[3]

Because of my wonderful personal experience with aerobics, I decided to produce a series for cable TV called "Aerobicise," which further changed my life. I followed soon after that with a syndicated television show called the ":20 Minute Workout." Three million men and women work out to my TV program five days a week.

It is now seven years since I attended that first aerobics class. I have bought and read every book on diet, exercise, life extension, toxins, vitamins, etc., that I could find, including hundreds of scientific papers. *Aerobicise* is a culmination of all that I now know about health and exercise.

In order to understand what had happened to my body, and what further changes were possible, I applied what I had learned from theoretical science to the tangible world of physiology. Since all of nature follows the same laws of the universe, I knew that if I cross-referenced the latest scientific and medical research, I would find significant intersections of the two disciplines. At those intersections would be the beginnings of an understanding of how the pieces of the puzzle of life fit together. That brought me to a number of interesting realizations about our bodies, our minds, and our behavior—and how inextricably interwoven they are.

We are the most highly evolved lifeform on earth. Our evolution is a result of billions of matings over billions of years. The process continues every day. Choices that each individual makes about whom to date and then mate with directly impact the human evolutionary chain.

In *The Evolution of Human Sexuality,* Donald Symons says that if we pass down a close approximation of our genetic code to the next generation, then we have succeeded as a species; if we do not reproduce, then we have failed as far as nature is concerned.[4] This new understanding of our biological motivations puts a different perspective on why we do what we do, including why we work out.

Having spent much of the last several years in health clubs in Los Angeles, I can tell you firsthand that the majority of the people who work out are between relationships. Usually, within days of finding a new companion, they stop coming to the club. Several months later, they inevitably show up again, noticeably fatter, having just broken up with their friend.

If you are like most of us, you are exercising to look better, so that you can get a mate. We will help you do that. If you are currently in a relationship, you must be prepared for your new fitness program to alter the relationship. Just as any change will affect the delicate balance of a relationship, so will your decision to be healthy.

Getting physically healthy is probably the most extensive personal change you can make, because what you really are doing is changing your attitude toward life. Your relationship can rebalance and be stronger than ever, or it can topple to the ground if your mate feels threatened by the new you. The important thing to remember is that you are doing this for yourself.

THE BIOLOGICAL IMPERATIVE

THE CATASTROPHE THEORY

Every living thing—plant or animal—is connected on the life chain. When one is affected, others will be too, often in opposing ways.

Basically, this theory holds that we evolve, and the world around us changes, through unaccountable catastrophes. If a drought hits your fields, for example, it might be devastating for you, but for the birds who feed on your unharvested seed, it would be a windfall. The next season would bring with it a bumper crop of birds. What's disastrous for one form of life can be a bonanza to another.

There are also less obvious catastrophes. A gentle breeze puts a strain on a tree that causes living cells within the tree to be stressed enough so that they are damaged. The tree responds by growing more cells, thereby becoming stronger through the catastrophe that has befallen it. The same might be said of exercise and the human body.

Think of exercise as the systematic tearing down of body cells so that a new generation of cells can grow strong. (A gardener might liken this phenomenon to pruning a plant, to encourage it to grow stronger and flower more often.) Body builders have understood this concept for years. They work out every other day—one day they tear down their tissue and the next day they let it grow back, bigger and stronger than it was.

If you don't want to look like a body builder, we recommend that you exercise six days a week, thereby tearing down the old, fatty tissue without giving the body time to build bulk, just enough time to build health.

HOW TO USE THIS BOOK

This book will teach you how to do the minimal amount of exercise you need each day in order to look younger longer and to be better prepared for change, since constant change is what life is all about.

Most health books are very one-sided, emphasizing a particular diet or exercise or food supplement. This is a balanced book: We will show you how the proper *combination* of exercise, food, and vitamins can keep you younger and more vigorous.

Aerobicise is designed with only one or two exercises per page to minimize confusion while you are working out. Two hundred beautiful photographs teach you how to do over 70 aerobic exercises.

Chapter 5 puts together a series of aerobics routines for quick reference. This chapter is broken down into 3-, 6-, 9-, 12-, 15-, 18-, and 21-minute workouts, so that once you are familiar with the individual exercises you only have a few pages to turn, making this book practical to use while exercising.

Chapter 6 includes special tone-up workouts for specific parts of your body. The exercises are grouped according to the part of the body that they benefit: arms, waist, stomach, buttocks, legs, and thighs.

The primary workouts start with three-minute routines, allowing rank beginners or the over-45 crowd to begin an exercise program safely. For those who want to work out for more than 21 minutes, the individual exercises can be done for longer periods of time. It's clear, though, that for good health, *12 minutes a day of aerobic exercise, six days a week, is all you really need to stay in shape.*

Aerobics is the only form of exercise we must have to live. ("Aerobic" refers to any organism that lives or is active only in the presence of oxygen, and that means us.) We increase our oxygen intake through aerobic exercise to purify our bodies of the toxins we eat. Exercise fads may come and go, but we can never do without aerobics.

And the best, most efficient kind of aerobic exercise is our Aerobicise program, which uses fast music to help you keep your exercise pace up —and to let you have fun by making you think you are dancing instead of working out.

CHAPTER ONE

IT'S NEVER TOO LATE

Weep not that the world changes—did it keep a stable, changeless state, 'twere cause indeed to weep.

—William Cullen Bryant,
"Mutation" (1824)

A journey of a thousand miles must begin with a single step.

—Lao-Tzu (c. 604–531 B.C.)

"You are what you think." "You are what you eat." Both statements are true. But the more important of the two is the first one, because when you change how you think, you will change what you eat.

Most people are afraid that if they change the way they think they will lose themselves. That fear is ungrounded. As a matter of fact, if we do not change the way we think, as we grow older we get more and more unhappy, and then we *do* lose ourselves. The world changes around us, so we must change, too, or we will be in the way of the next generation, and our old-fashioned ways will make us unhappy and hasten our departure.

We can stay around if we keep a young outlook on life and can help the next generation grow stronger. Doing this will prolong our lives and give them meaning.

We truly are as young as we feel, and if we think young and socialize with young people, we will feel young. Most old people are around other old and dying people, and use their behavior patterns as an excuse for their own laziness. Instead, you must look around for the exceptions who excel above the norm for your age group, and follow their example. Ronald Reagan, George Burns, Bob Hope, Jack LaLanne, Lee Iacocca, Linus Pauling, Jane Fonda, Geraldine Ferraro, Katharine Hepburn, and other equally vital business leaders, government officials, professionals, scientists, entertainers, and artists should be your inspiration. You can slow the aging process and feel years younger, if you follow the easy steps in this book.

Movement is change, and change is life. Yet we are taught to stand still: Society's interests are best served if we stay on the same job, with the same mate and in the same house, so that our institutions and governments can keep track of us. I feel that the false sense of security we gain from being stable (not changing) is counterproductive to the way our bodies were programmed to thrive. It is through instability that we move forward and grow. Our lives are enriched by change, by risks taken, new people and fresh ideas experienced.

Change is initially frightening, and the more insecure you are, the more threatening it is. Once you make the break with your past and start to move forward, though, you will soon find that change is invigorating—and then, essential.

People seek comfort. The familiar is comfortable to us, so our lives become routinized, full of recognizable patterns. This is fine, if the patterns we're talking about are the traditions of celebrating happy events and reinforcing positive symbols, but it can be very bad if the patterns in your life are ruts of negative, self-destructive behavior.

Being irresponsible about your body is a negative, self-destructive life pattern that's very easy to fall into. How comfortable does that really feel to you? My guess is that it no longer feels good, that you are ready for *change*, or you wouldn't be reading this book.

EXCUSES WE USE NOT TO EXERCISE

The old excuses just don't make it: "I have a bad back, bad knees, arthritis." "I'll do it after the holiday/vacation/summer/winter/Johnny goes to school/my new job is under control." "I don't have time." "The health club is too expensive, too far away." (As you'll see, these last two excuses are totally inapplicable to the Aerobicise program.) You can always find a new reason to put off getting in shape. Now is the time to *stop* making excuses and start taking action.

GIVING UP DEPENDENCIES

It's not easy to change the way you think, to change what you value and how you live your life. To do so, you must give up a lot of dependencies, emotional and physical dependencies.

You are probably emotionally dependent on food, too much of it and the wrong kind. You are also likely to be dependent on your lazy, unhealthy lifestyle. Even though it doesn't feel so great anymore, it is what you are used to, and changing it is scary.

Furthermore, you may be physically dependent on drugs: cigarettes, alcohol, stimulants, tranquilizers, pain medications, marijuana, or cocaine, all of which fill strong emotional needs as well.

It is time to give up these dependencies, time to be *independent*—time to get the monkey off your back.

How do you know where to start? There is such a plethora of diet/exercise/self-actualization formulas out there that it is very difficult to know whom to believe.

Don't use this profusion of information as another excuse to stall action. Sure, there will always be new information on the horizon, but you can educate yourself well enough now to be able to evaluate it intelligently when it comes along.

That's what I did, after I realized that no one had as serious an interest in my health as I did. Because I am an ordinary person, a person who spent most of his life being overweight, smoking and drinking and not exercising, the method for getting and staying in shape that worked for me can work for you.

I am not an athlete or a movie star who can spend hours a day with a private workout instructor, or a doctor who has a vested interest in the party line of the medical profession. This book is written for people like me. It contains all the currently available information that you really need to get fit. If I could do it, you can do it.

Your mind-set is everything. You must cross the critical border between thinking that it would be nice to be thin and healthy (but continuing your bad habits and hating yourself for it) and deciding that you are unhappy with your body and your life *and are going to change.*

Remember, life is fluid, always moving forward. In order to be part of life, people must open up to change. You will not disappear, but will transform into the vital, vigorous person waiting inside you right now. If you aren't moving forward, you are dying.

You can start on your way toward fitness today, by taking small, manageable steps. Don't be intimidated. All you need is the will to change.

CHAPTER TWO

WHERE'S THE FAT?

Gluttony is an emotional escape, a sign something is eating us.

—Peter De Vries

Imprisoned in every fat man a thin one is wildly signalling to be let out.

—Cyril Connolly

Fat is the enemy. The amount of harm that will come to you from eating fat is thousands of times greater than from any other food substance or man-made toxin.[1]

If you give up eating fat, and start exercising, you will slim down and probably stay healthy and young-looking longer. You can keep your body thinking it is young and healthy, thereby prolonging your vital years. And that will make you less likely to get cancer, hardening of the arteries, and other diseases of the aged.

What Is Fat?

The dietary category "fat" includes what we commonly think of as fats: butter, margarine, mayonnaise, lard, and other solid fats. It also includes oils: vegetable, peanut, olive oils, etc. Fat is also present, but less obvious, in such foods as eggs, cheese, whole milk, meats, nuts, and seeds.[2]

There is so much fat available in your diet, in fact, that it is *impossible* to get too little of it, even if you cut out everything you can think of that contains fat.[3] *You can get your entire day's requirement of fat from one large bowl of oatmeal.*[4] (See chart on page 213 for the fat content of over 325 foods.)

Since most of us eat *far* more fat than that supplied in a tablespoon of half-and-half (whole milk at breakfast, butter on our toast, mayonnaise on our tuna sandwich at lunch, salad dressing at dinner, a "well-marbled" steak, sour cream on our baked potato, ice cream for dessert), we are overdosing on a deadly substance—one which offers precious little in return for its potential harm.

The average American's diet consists of about 45% fat, 20% protein, and 35% carbohydrates.[5] As you'll see, this formula is very unhealthy. What you won't see here is another numerical formula to replace the above. Most of the so-called health and diet books tell you exactly what percentage you should have from each food group every day, and then go on to list sample menus with weights and measurements of portions. Come on, how many people are going to carry those pages around and pull them out along with a scale and a measuring cup at restaurants or at a dinner party?

The *only* way you will learn to eat right and be healthy is by understanding the concepts behind a healthful diet, and then by applying your own common sense to your eating patterns. Our "formula" is very simple: Just cut down as much as possible on the foods that are bad for you (fat), and increase your intake of the foods that are good (fiber—

more on that soon; also see chart on fiber content of common foods, page 219.)

Go for the big picture: don't allow yourself to avoid the major changes you should be making by preoccupying yourself with counting minuscule amounts of salt or sugar—neither one of which is likely to do you any serious harm unless you eat huge quantities of them.

THE KILLER FAT

Excess fat kills us three ways: by destroying our ability to metabolize food efficiently, causing us to create our own excess body fat and health problems attendant to being overweight; by shutting down the amount of oxygen our blood can carry to the brain and muscles (ever wonder why people fall asleep after a heavy meal?); and by clogging our arteries with cholesterol, which manifests itself in gout and hardening of the arteries, the latter culminating in heart attacks.[6]

A diet high in fat has also been linked to a greater incidence of cancer of the colon, breast, prostate, ovaries, and rectum.[7] In fact, a paper presented in 1985 by a group of renowned doctors documents a noteworthy increase in gallbladder, colon, prostate, rectum, and breast cancer (in addition to other diseases) in people who are just 20% overweight. (Previously, the medical community used 40% as the danger point.[8]) Fat in the diet is most likely what made those 20-percenters overweight.

The central function of fat is to provide energy, and since fat is a lightweight, compact form of calories, the body has evolved its internal storage system to stockpile fat. Because plants don't need the mobility we animals do, they store their energy in the heavier, bulkier form of carbohydrates.[9]

Fat has evolved into such a major energy supply that it is capable of providing the body with twice as many calories per pound as carbohydrates can.[10] Further, fat can be made from any other category of food; the body has been so sold on the efficiency and reliability of fat that it knows how to turn both protein and carbohydrates into fat once they get inside the system.[11]

The system by which the body converts food into energy is called the Kreb's Cycle, which operates only under *aerobic* conditions. In this cycle, everything that you put into your mouth comes together to be burned, recycled, stored, or modified according to your body's needs. The Kreb's Cycle readily makes fat from everything you eat or drink, with very few exceptions, such as salt and water.[12]

This would all be terrific, *if* we were still hunter-gatherers, roaming around the countryside looking for nuts and grasses to eat, supplementing our diets with a bird or a deer once a month. Unfortunately, our energy storage system is still operating under the premise that it might not get another acorn for four hours (hence, it wants *every* calorie, which means converting your food into fat for optimum storage). That leaves the average person with a serious fat overload.

Short of living on salt and water, what can you do to inspire your **KING** Kreb's Cycle to burn the fat you eat, and not to produce more fat from **CARBOHYDRATE** everything else? *Eat carbohydrates,* those "starches" that were anathema to your mother and doctors. Not only are carbohydrates 50% lower per pound in calories than fat, and generally contain a very high percentage of water, they are the only "clean-burning" fuel—they give off no toxins. They also produce the food that feeds the brain: blood sugar, called glucose.

Most surprisingly, *carbohydrates burn fat*. The easiest way to remember this critical concept is with the following catch phrase: Fat burns in the flame of carbohydrates.

The Kreb's Cycle can burn fat cleanly and effectively only when carbohydrates are present in the system. Carbohydrates are the kindling for the firewood of fat.[13]

There are two kinds of carbohydrates: simple and complex. You want the latter.

Simple carbohydrates are recognizable because they usually taste sweet: Sugar, honey, and syrups are all simple carbohydrates. Simple carbohydrates are also found in beer, milk, and milk products. They provide little nutritive value and are less filling than complex carbohydrates. They promote dental cavities in children and they stimulate your body to make fat by creating insulin, too much of which both activates fat production and makes you feel hungry.

Complex carbohydrates (also known as fiber)—found in pasta, enriched breads, potatoes, grains, cereals, vegetables, and fruits—will give your body the best possible nutrition for the least intake of calories. These foods will do nearly all your body's work for you, make you feel full and satisfied, ward off health problems you're likely to get if you let your diet be taken over by fats or animal and dairy protein, and *cause you no weight gain*. In fact, the best way to *lose* weight is on a high-complex-carbohydrate diet, combined with exercise.[14]

You can't go wrong with complex carbohydrates.

What about protein in all this? Isn't *that* what you are supposed to eat the most of to be slim and healthy? *No.*

Certainly your body needs protein, to build and repair bones, teeth, and tissue, but it does not need as much protein as an average American consumes each day. Excess protein in your diet will convert into fat, inhibit fat burning, cause the body to use muscle instead of fat for fuel (just the opposite of what you want) and dehydrate you.[15]

The body has no mechanism for storing extra protein; it must convert it into fat or glucose. So, eating a lot of protein will *not* build muscle, as commonly believed.[16] And because fat burns in the flame of carbohydrates, a diet that is high in protein is cheating your body of its kindling wood—carbohydrates. The protein you are eating is taking up space that should be going to carbohydrates, and is inhibiting efficient burning of fats for energy.

You don't want to convert protein into either fat or glucose, either. Your body certainly does not need any more fat than it already has, and glucose should be coming from carbohydrates.

Moreover, if you are on a high-protein, low-calorie diet in order to lose weight, your body will begin to "eat" its own flesh. Again, this is because you have limited your intake of carbohydrates. In this case, the protein you eat is needed immediately to make glucose for the brain (since there are no carbohydrates to do the job), and it cannot take care of the task for which it was meant—to repair and build tissues that have broken down since you last ate. Consequently, the muscles break down and are not repaired.[17]

(The same principle applies to fasting, which should be avoided. Because you do not have any carbohydrates to light a fire under the fat your cells have stored, you will not be able to burn off the fat. Therefore, you will not lose fat but will lose muscle, as your body converts its own body protein to glucose. A prolonged fast is devastating to your body muscle.[18])

Dehydration is yet another of the effects of protein overconsumption. When the body has used up all the protein it needs to do its repair work, it sends the excess to the liver, where it is converted into fat.

The negative effects of this are twofold: one, you wind up with more fat; two, the conversion process creates a very toxic by-product, ammonia, which in turn is quickly transformed into urea. Urea is fairly toxic, and so must be diluted in urine and released from the body. This is part of the normal physiological process, as long as you don't create too much. If you do, the body will need tremendous amounts of water to dilute it. No matter how much water you guzzle, a high-protein diet will leave your body thirsting for more. So it will suck the water it needs from its own tissues, leaving you dangerously dehydrated.[19]

Of course, we *do* need protein to do the construction and repair work while the carbohydrates supply the fuel. The question is where to get the best kind.

Here's where we come upon another surprise: Amino acids, protein's "building blocks," are best obtained *not* from red meat (which contains a very high percentage of fat), nor from dairy products (ditto), but from grains, roots, vegetables, and fruits—and that means pasta, rice, breads, potatoes, beans, and apples. Yes, *carbohydrates*, complex carbohydrates, preferably in an unrefined, minimally processed form.[20]

It's certainly okay to eat some meat, as long as you try to keep it lean, and some dairy products, which should be low-fat (even better, nonfat) whenever possible, and some eggs (try not to cook them in too much butter). But the more you stick to complex carbohydrates for your protein, the better off you'll be.

NEGATIVE VIBES

If you watch television, you know that the fat guy is always the bad guy or the comic and never the hero, certainly never the romantic lead. The same kind of double standard applies in real life. It is definitely the thin people in our society who have the greatest opportunities. Their attractiveness opens doors and promotes them above their fat counterparts.

If it is so obvious that being fat is a serious disadvantage, why do people have so much trouble eating the right foods and getting in shape? Because they are being sabotaged by their own neuroses.

I once had an advertising client whose wife weighed at least 250 pounds. We were in Portugal on a shooting for men's clothing. Over dinner one evening, the woman volunteered that the reason she was so fat was so that she didn't have to deal with being "hit on"—by strangers and by her own husband. I was amazed at the time by how astute she was and I wondered if other fat people were as aware of why they are fat.

Because we all know that in our culture fat is considered unattractive and undesirable, being fat is being antisocial. When you are fat, you are sending off nonverbal signals to tell other people to keep their distance —literally. You are pushing people out of intimacy range and letting them know that you are not interested in having intercourse on any level, particularly sexual. Fat is the best possible suit of armor to shield yourself against amorous pursuit.

The unfortunate implications of being fat are that you are usually very angry, because no one pays you much attention (at least not the kind of attention you *claim* to want). And so you seek solace in the dependable comfort of a friend who always comes through for you, who always makes you feel good—food. And you get fatter, and are further rejected socially, and so on and so on.

Until you have had enough, until you decide that it's time to change your life.

THROW AWAY YOUR BATHROOM SCALE

The first thing you need to do is to *forget about how much you weigh.* It is not how many pounds comprise your body weight but what those pounds are made up of that counts. There are plenty of temporarily "thin" people who don't weigh much—and who are out of shape, flabby and, yes, *fat.* They are "fat" because their bodies are made up of a higher proportion of fat to muscle than they should be. They don't necessarily weigh "too much" because fat weighs less than muscle. But they are on their way to being both overfat *and* overweight.[21]

For example, look at what happens to people as they age. As you get older and more out of shape, muscles atrophy and are invaded by fat. But you don't register any extra pounds when you stand on the scale, for the fat is lighter than the muscle it has replaced. That is, until your muscle degeneration slows down. Then you begin to deposit fat outside the muscle and you will start to gain weight.[22]

Your goal should be to increase your muscle and decrease your fat, to become physically fit. If you are within a normal weight range, this may actually cause you to "gain weight"—that is, you may weigh a few more pounds because muscle is heavier than fat. But you will look sleek and firm, be healthy, and feel terrific. That is what we are talking about here —looking, feeling, and *being* healthy, not weighing in at some arbitrary "perfect" weight.

AND THE FAT GET FATTER

Sixty to 70% of the energy that your muscles need to operate when the body is at rest comes from fat. Storage of fat is, therefore, natural and necessary for survival. The problem for fat people is that they are storing too much fat and not burning it off.

Fat people are making more fat all the time, *while eating less than thin people.* How can that be? It's because the fat person's body has lost its ability to convert fat to fuel and to burn it off. And the fatter you get, the lower the rate at which you can use your fat. So once you become fat, you get quickly locked into a fat-producing cycle, and one peanut butter and jelly sandwich will take you a day to metabolize, while your thin friend will burn it off in three hours and be ready for a pizza.

Once you understand why you have been unable to lose weight, why those diets and spot-reducing plans have never worked, you'll be able to begin your journey toward being thin.

There are two reasons why you want your body to convert fat to muscle: Muscle uses 90% of your calories, even when you are not moving; and a certain kind of enzyme, which lives only in the muscles, can raise calorie use fiftyfold when you *are* exercising. It's quite clear, then, that if you want to burn more calories, you need more muscle to do it.

The calorie-consuming enzymes inside your muscle cells are proteins, very delicate proteins. People who are in the process of getting fit are building more and more of these enzymes every day; people whose bodies are atrophying are slowly discarding theirs. The fat are getting ever fatter, while the fit are on a one-way street toward greater fitness.

Another reason fat people favor more fat production is rooted in a phenomenon called insulin insensitivity. The fat person's cells do not know how to process their own insulin, which should be acting as the doorman to the cells when glucose comes knocking. Glucose (blood sugar, the brain's food) wants to lodge in the muscle cells for storage, but it can't, so it floats around waiting for the impaired insulin to open the cells' doors. The wait is so long that much of it finds a home in the cells of which the fat person has the most—fat cells.

Once inside the fat cells, glucose changes into fat. Yet again, the fat person is creating more of what he or she needs least—more fat.[23]

NO MORE DIETS

Extreme diets are not going to get you where you want to be. Certainly, if you are overweight, you should cut back on overall food consumption. The *only* thing that will turn you into a healthy eater and keep you one is to change your eating patterns for good, not just until your "diet" is over.

Again, the most important thing to do is to *get rid of fats.* The easiest way to do this is to stay away from fried foods, sauces and gravies, cold cuts, hot dogs, bacon, large meat portions, and rich desserts. Restricting the amount of butter, margarine, cheese, mayonnaise, salad dressing, and eggs in your diet is also a good idea. Never worry about getting too little of anything in this category. You cannot get less fat than you need.

You need not become a fanatic to make a healthy eating program work. You can still go out to restaurants and share meals with friends. You can adjust what you eat one day to accommodate what you ate the day (or meal) before. Just use your own good judgment. If you go to an Italian restaurant, order pasta with fresh tomato sauce instead of cream sauce and sorbet in place of zabaglione for dessert. You can even eat things that aren't good for you every once in a while, too—a little bit of anything, even the world's richest chocolate cake, isn't going to kill you.

Avoid limiting yourself to one meal a day. This creates a 23-hour "fast." If you spread the same amount of calories out over five or six small meals, you will put less stress on your body and keep the weight you lose off.

Your body reacts to fasting as an emergency, so it starts to store all the fuel—fat—it can, in case there is no more coming for a very long time. If you continue to fool your body into thinking it is always on the brink of starvation, it will become very adept at making and storing fat and will continue to do so when you go off your diet. You will probably gain more weight back than if you had treated your body decently and spread your calories out.[24]

Once you get tough with your will power in order to lose weight, you will find that as soon as you are stabilized at a healthy weight, your appetite will control the amount of food you need all by itself. Once you are in touch with your body through eating right and exercise, it will tell you when it needs food and when it doesn't. It will even tell you what *kind* of food it needs. You will no longer want rich, fatty foods—as impossible as that may seem. You will actually crave a crisp, juicy apple instead of a gooey chocolate-chip cookie. (Most of the time. When you occasionally want that cookie, have one. No point in being a martyr.)

Vitamins

Do you need vitamins to supplement your diet? *Yes.* You'd have to eat as much as the Dallas Cowboys to get all the vitamins and minerals you need. It's much better to get them in capsule form and to forgo all those extra calories. There is nothing a "natural" vitamin or mineral obtained directly from food can do that one bought at a reputable pharmacy, market, or health-food store can't.

Please note that although I recommend taking vitamins from a bottle, I *do not* recommend taking drugs or popping aspirins all day long. Vitamins that come from a bottle are good for you; almost every other kind of pill that comes in one is not.

$$220 - 30 = 190 \quad 190 \times .75 = 142.5.$$

That figure (rounded off)—142—is your target heart rate. If you reach that figure during 12 minutes of exercise, six days a week, you will receive maximum aerobic conditioning.

WHY TWELVE MINUTES

There seems to be something special about doing 12 minutes of exercise per day, six days a week. More experts have used this number than any other. This does not mean two six-minute exercise periods with a rest in between. It means 12 minutes of continuous aerobics.

Use the following chart so that you may work up to your 12 minutes of aerobics per day. (The seven fitness levels listed here correspond to the categories for the workouts you'll be using.) If you wish to increase your exercise past 12 minutes per day you may, but for the average person, who is not trying to be an athlete, there is no need to. There is less benefit from the next 12 minutes and more likelihood of injury.[6]

We strongly recommend that you do not wear extra weights or carry weights in your hands when you work out. Putting any extra strain on your body increases the chance of injuries and slows you down. If you want a body builder's body, go to the nearest gym and work out with the body builders. Your chances of being injured are much less if you are working out under their supervision.

MINUTES OF EXERCISES PER DAY (6 DAYS A WEEK)

	WARM-UP	AEROBIC	COOL-DOWN	TOTAL
VERY OUT OF SHAPE	1	1	1	3
OUT OF SHAPE	2	3	1	6
GETTING IN SHAPE	2	5	2	9
IN SHAPE	2	8	2	12
GREAT SHAPE	3	10	2	15
FABULOUS SHAPE	3	12	3	18
IN TRAINING	4	14	3	21

WHAT EXERCISES ARE AEROBIC?

Only exercises that are done fast enough to raise your heartbeat to 80% of its maximum are aerobic. This will vary, of course, on the shape you are in. A person who is very out of shape may get his or her heartbeat into an aerobic state by walking up one flight of stairs; an athlete might have to run for ten minutes before his or her heartbeat reaches an aerobic level.[7]

Since your heartbeat increases at different rates during different exercises—and nothing is as efficient as our Aerobicise program, not even running—you must work out much longer at other exercises to gain the equivalent of twelve minutes of Aerobicise.

AEROBICISE IS FUN

According to *Shape* magazine, there are 18.7 million Americans reaping the benefits of aerobic exercise. It's more than the desire for fitness that keeps these millions of people going back to it every day: They are having a good time.

It is critical that you actually *like* exercising, otherwise you will never *continue* to exercise. The enjoyment factor is another reason to try our Aerobicise program—it's so much fun that you'll look forward to doing it.

The key to our Aerobicise program is music. Fast, loud music energizes you, keeps you going longer at a steadier pace, and makes working out less tedious—more like dancing.

You can see from the following how the most well-known aerobic exercises stack up against Aerobicise. They are divided into four categories: exercises requiring 12 minutes, 15 minutes, 30 minutes, and 40 minutes of steady activity. You may want to use some of these activities for variety, or because they are nice for socializing or for enjoying the outdoors, but remember: None is as effective as the Aerobicise routines for quick, overall conditioning.

T W E L V E   M I N U T E S

jumping rope

running in place to music

aerobics classes

Lifecycle (stationary bicycle)

F I F T E E N   M I N U T E S

jogging/running

cross-country skiing

rowing

mini-trampoline

T H I R T Y   M I N U T E S

walking

outdoor bicycling on a flat path (no coasting
allowed)

F O R T Y   M I N U T E S

swimming

JUMPING ROPE:

The equipment required for jumping rope is a soft surface (a soft carpet remnant), a jump rope that reaches just about to nipple height when you stand on it with both feet, and some good, loud music. Start your music at 105 beats per minute, and increase as your fitness level increases (see Chapter 7, "Loud Music").

Instead of alternating feet, jump with both feet to decrease the trauma on your legs and feet (you will be dividing the impact of your weight in two). If your target heart rate can't be reached with this formula, speed up the music.

RUNNING IN PLACE TO MUSIC:

One of the benefits of running in place as an exercise is that it can be adjusted to suit your fitness level: The fit person will use very fast music and lift the legs high to get the heartbeat up to training level, while the severely out of shape can start out with a fairly slow beat and may need do no more than raise the heels to get an aerobic effect.

AEROBICS CLASSES:

The way to tell that you have found a good aerobics class is the length of the line you have to wait in to get in and the number of bodies packed into the room. Remember, you do not need to take the whole class. (If you do, you are probably in competition with your ego.) Stay for the aerobics, and then leave, for most of the other exercises are "spot reducers." (Since they have no ability to reduce anything, they would be better named "spot builders.") Aerobics is the only form of exercise that will burn fat. There are no short cuts.

LIFECYCLE:

This is the state-of-the-art stationary bicycle. Unlike those that came before it, the Lifecycle actually alters pedal resistance to give you a warm-up and a cool-down phase, and to create a landscape of hills and straightaways designed to give you an efficient aerobic workout. Its onboard computer controls resistance, shows you your pedaling speed, elapsed time, and calories-per-hour consumption rate. Twelve programs are available to match your personal level of fitness; advanced cyclists can access a *million* predesigned rides by selecting the "random" program, making it impossible to get bored.

If you use the Lifecycle correctly, it is possible to give your cardiovascular system a workout that will get your heart rate up into the target range.[8]

JOGGING/RUNNING:

Currently the most popular aerobic exercise, jogging/running is easy to begin (very little skill is required), inexpensive, completely portable (there is always some ground you can cover outside), and burns fat very quickly. The only thing you need is a good pair of running shoes.

The down side of running lies in the injuries that can occur if you do not warm up properly, do not wear the correct shoes, or if you run excessive distances (25 miles or more per week). People with weak backs or knees should try to run on grass or dirt as often as possible, to cushion stressful impact. (Exercises to strengthen the stomach and quadriceps, which support the back and knees, respectively, should begin *before* taking up running—and Aerobicise—if these are problem areas.)

The up side of the pounding you take in running is that the bones and joints actually tend to get thicker and stronger due to the pressure exerted on them. This can protect them against osteoporosis, the deterioration of the bones that occurs with aging, and is often brought on by menopause. The same applies to our Aerobicise program.

What does not apply to Aerobicise is the uneven pace at which you often exercise while jogging/running. Because you tend naturally to slow down occasionally (even if you run on a track, but particularly if you run on the obstacle course of the streets), you do not keep your heart rate at a consistent level. With Aerobicise, the music keeps you moving quickly and evenly, and there are no people, cars, dogs, or potholes to dodge. Even if you could run at a smooth pace, you probably wouldn't be running at the number of beats per minute you need for maximum aerobic benefit.

CROSS-COUNTRY SKIING:

This utilizes more muscles in the upper body than running does, and the more muscles you involve in your exercise, the greater the aerobic benefit to the whole body.

Other advantages are that cross-country skiing is usually done at high altitudes and in cold weather, both of which contribute to a tougher workout.

Of course, cross-country skiing has a very obvious drawback: It's highly seasonal, and requires expensive equipment and some skill. It is also one of the most enjoyable of exercises, to which anyone who has reveled in a graceful glide through a snow-laden forest will happily attest. Because it is so much fun (and so much fun to do with friends), you tend to get in much more than your fifteen minutes—a bonus that can easily be used to justify that snack you brought along on your back.

ROWING:

An indoor rowing machine is an expensive investment, but it can provide good aerobic exercise. A good machine will utilize almost all the major muscles—in your arms, back, abdomen, and legs. (It is important to get one with a seat that slides back and forth so you can push with your legs.)

MINI-TRAMPOLINE:

The mini-trampoline is just large enough for a person to run in place. While the mini-trampoline is probably to be recommended for people with serious bone and/or muscle problems (because its elastic surface reduces trauma), it does not offer as high a conditioning level as our Aerobicise program, jogging, or even running in place. This is because the trampoliner's legs spring back up without any energy expenditure. And since the real world does not take place on a trampoline, the muscles you use trampolining are not the same you need in a normal lifestyle. You also do not get the bone-strengthening benefit that you would get from our Aerobicise workout.

WALKING:

THIRTY MINUTES

Walking has the portability and low-cost attributes of running without the trauma to the knees and joints. However, if you are either young or in good shape, you may have to simulate that odd, elbows-akimbo "race walker" style that allows you to walk very fast in order to get to the aerobic, fat-burning level of running. For the elderly or the out of shape, walking at a normal rate will drive the pulse rate up to an aerobic level.

Walking is particularly attractive to people who feel embarrassed about running in public. After a few months of a serious walking program, those same people who wouldn't be caught running down the street without a disguise will most likely have sped up their pace to a jog, and soon, to a run.

Again, though, you are unlikely to be able to get your heartbeat up to Aerobicise levels and to keep it there for 12 straight minutes. So, like the rest of these sports, fast walking is not a substitute for the quick, fun efficiency of Aerobicise, but rather is to be used as an occasional variant or supplement.

Of course, you *must* actually *walk,* and it must be both fast and steady. Window shopping is not aerobic exercise.

OUTDOOR BICYCLING:

Because cycling is a "non-weight bearing" exercise, it is especially well suited to overweight or older people. In fact, cyclists in general seem to suffer less from the wear and tear on muscles and joints than runners do.

There is no optimum speed necessary for aerobic benefit, so if you want to go slowly but have geared *down,* your cardiovascular system will be getting just as good a workout as if you were pedaling in a higher gear and going much faster. The only measurement that counts is your heartbeat rate—just get it up to your target rate and keep it there. (If you are in a low gear on your 10- or 15-speed bike, your legs will be going fast even though you are traversing the ground slowly.)

Equipment can be kept to a minimum: a good bicycle (investing in a 15-speed is definitely worth the extra dollars, because the smoothness of the changes from hills to valleys to straightaways keeps your heart pumping at a steadier pace) and a good helmet.

The drawback to cycling is in finding a good route, that is, one long enough to require no stopping. For, once again, you won't be able to get your heart pumping and keep it pumping at the Aerobicise level unless your exercise is steady.

Luckily, I have easy access to a nearly level bike path (no stoplights) that runs 17 miles along the Southern California coastline, and so am able to ride most weekends from Venice Beach to Redondo Beach and back—26 miles of even terrain, with a gorgeous view and sunshine and fresh air to boot. Midwesterners might be able to find a flat path of considerable length, but most other folks will be hard pressed to come up with a bicycling route that will provide the even ground and continuous ride that is necessary for aerobic bicycling.

Remember: Coasting is cheating.

SWIMMING:

Because it uses all the major muscles in the body, swimming will limber up your arms and legs and give you more total conditioning than most other forms of exercise, but you must swim *extremely* fast to get your heart rate up to an aerobic level. For a person swimming at an advanced level, then, the sport can provide good aerobic exercise: the

FORTY
MINUTES

average swimmer will have a very hard time gaining the necessary speed.

Swimming is a nontraumatic sport: the water's buoyancy reduces pressure on joints and bones. Swimmers can log up to 10 miles a day without exposing themselves to great danger with muscle pulls or joint trauma. Compared with running, that's a significant benefit for those with bone and/or muscle problems.

A steady program, though, contains its own set of unique problems: chlorine-damaged hair, dried-out skin, those nagging ear-eye-sinus infections, not to mention the occasional vaginal infection picked up from a public pool. (The only way to guard against the latter is by choosing your pool for high hygiene level and low population level.) And, of course, there are the obvious drawbacks: You must either have a pool in your backyard or drive to get to one; and the amount of time it takes to wash and style your hair every time you want to exercise makes it pretty impractical on a daily basis.

You cannot expect to burn fat through a program that relies solely on swimming, either. An Aerobicise (or a runner's) body will shed as much weight as it can in order to increase speed and agility; a swimmer's body likes to conserve its fat in order to provide warmth and buoyancy (just look at a gazelle's body next to a sea lion's).[9]

AEROBICISE BENEFITS

The following benefits will accrue to anyone who becomes aerobically fit, which can most easily be accomplished by practicing our Aerobicise routines six days a week for 12 minutes a day. They are so extensive that you will actually feel that your life has changed drastically for the better. And it will have.

Our Aerobicise program will:

• Help you lose weight: Aerobic exercise is the only form of exercise that will burn fat. Coupled with a change in your diet, this will speed up your metabolism, so that you burn fat at a higher rate all the time, whether you are washing the dishes or working at a desk. For the most significant change in metabolism, work out in the morning: You will burn fat and experience the emotional and psychological benefits of aerobics for the remainder of the day. Don't forget, though, that weight loss is only of importance to people who are truly overweight. The rest of us should be concerned with losing *fat*, not weight.

• Give you more energy: Because aerobics will increase your metabolic rate, you will feel more energetic—in fact, you will *be* more energetic. You will lose that sluggish feeling that hits when energy is low, and

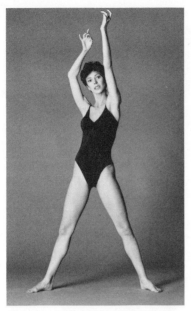

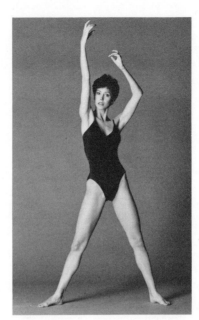

3

Side
Stretches

Stand; feet shoulder width apart and slightly turned out; stomach held in and hips tucked under. Bring both arms up to your head. Reach up with your LEFT arm 2 counts, feeling the stretch in your LEFT side.

Reach up with your RIGHT arm 2 counts. Stretch up and out from the rib cage. Then, single counts LEFT and RIGHT. Stretch it long.

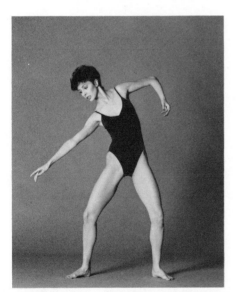

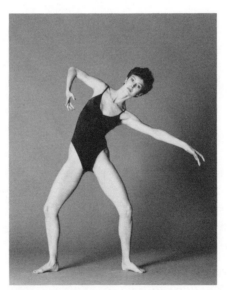

4

Bow &
Arrow

Stand with feet shoulder width apart; weight even over both feet; knees slightly bent; stomach held in and hips tucked under. Starting to the RIGHT, reach RIGHT arm out straight as left arm bows up. Feel the stretch in your LEFT side. Come back to center.

Then reach LEFT arm out straight as RIGHT arm bows up. Be sure to pull directly to the side, keeping your body front at all times. Single counts RIGHT and LEFT.

GENERIC EXERCISES FOR THE AEROBICISE WORKOUTS   51

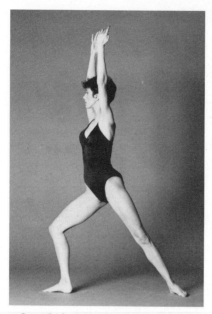

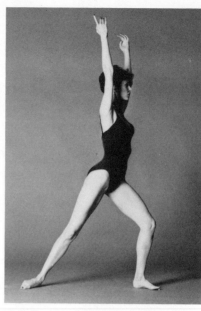

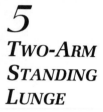

5
TWO-ARM STANDING LUNGE

Stand with feet wide apart; arms at sides. Lunge body and RIGHT leg to the RIGHT as both arms swing up above your head. You should feel the stretch from your calves up through your arms. This is a great overall stretch and should be done with speed and fluidity to get the most aerobic benefit.

Briefly come center with arms at your sides. Then, lunge to the LEFT. Keep it fluid. Use your arms for momentum.

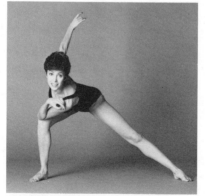

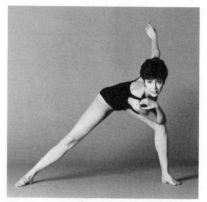

6
ELBOW-TO-KNEE LUNGE

Stand with feet twice your shoulder width apart. With a flat back, lunge to the RIGHT, reaching LEFT elbow to RIGHT knee and let your RIGHT arm swing up behind toward the ceiling.

Reverse to the LEFT, reaching RIGHT elbow to LEFT knee in single counts. Keep your stomach muscles in and breathe out as you lunge RIGHT and LEFT.

7
TOE
TOUCHES

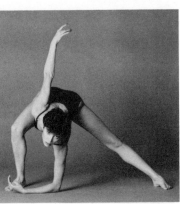

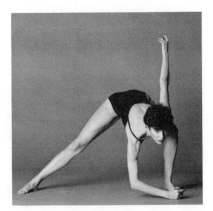

With feet twice your shoulder width apart, lunge to the RIGHT, reaching LEFT elbow to the floor as your RIGHT arm swings up toward the ceiling.

Then, lunge to the LEFT, reaching RIGHT elbow to the floor as LEFT arm swings up toward the ceiling. Reach down as far as you can. Keep your back flat and your stomach muscles held in.

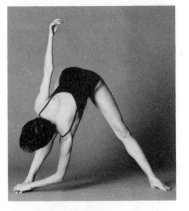

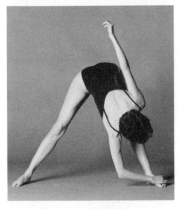

Straighten your legs and alternate reaching LEFT hand to RIGHT foot . . .

. . . and RIGHT hand to LEFT foot. Let your other arm swing up behind you. Single counts.

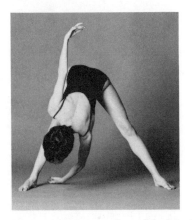

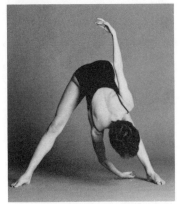

Now, reach LEFT hand behind RIGHT foot . . .

. . . and RIGHT hand behind LEFT foot in single counts. Pull out of the spine, keeping your back as straight as possible.

8 FLAT 2 PUSH THROUGH

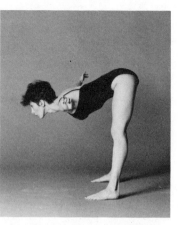

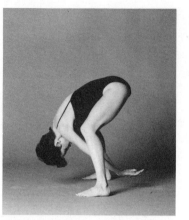

Stand with feet a little more than shoulder width apart. Your back is flat and your arms are out parallel to the ground. Gently pulse your back toward the floor 2 counts.

Then, bend your knees and push your hands and head through your legs 2 counts. Keep your stomach muscles in and breathe out as you push through.

9 STANDING STRETCH

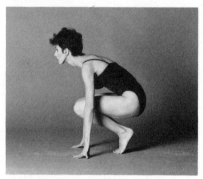

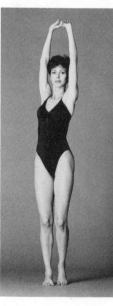

Bring your feet together and hands on the floor in front of you.

Gently roll up to a standing position with your hands above your head. With palms toward the ceiling, push your arms up and slightly back. Feel the stretch in your arms, shoulders, and upper back. Stretch it out and breathe.

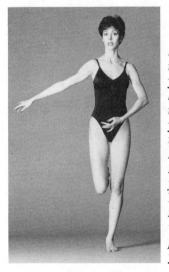

10 JOG

Stand straight with feet together. Begin by picking up your feet lightly. Land on the balls of your feet and work it through the heels. Pressing your heels to the floor takes the strain off the front of your legs. Keep it loose. Keep it light. Let your arms swing freely across your body. Remember: If you find any move too difficult along the way, just take it to an easy jog and keep going as long as you can.

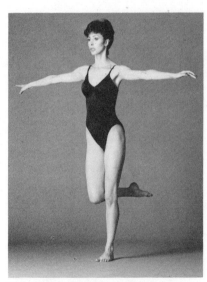

11 JOG/ARM CIRCLES

Feet jog in place. Arms out at shoulder height. Circle arms front with palms down 4 counts. Circle back with palms up 4 counts. Keep those stomach muscles tight and breathe out. Be sure to pull up out of the torso, and keep your shoulders down.

12 JOG/PUSH FRONT

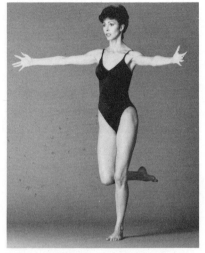

Jog. Arms out at shoulder height. Arms push front with palms front 4 counts . . .

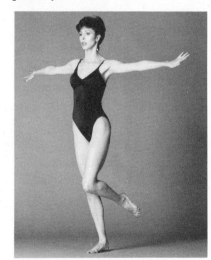

. . . then arms push back with palms back 4 counts. Be sure to keep your arms up (letting them fall below shoulder height is not giving you the maximum benefit to your arm muscles). If your arms get tired, shake them out then put them back up and keep going.

13
Jog/Hands To Shoulders

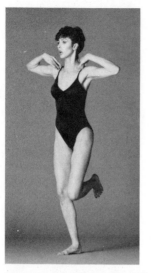

Jog. Arms out at shoulder height. Keep your upper arms still as you bring your hands to your shoulders . . .

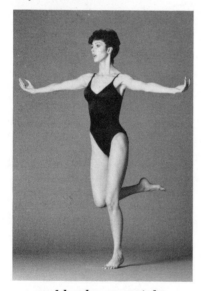

. . . and back out straight. This is good for your triceps, the muscles on the back of your upper arms.

14
Jog/ Reach Up

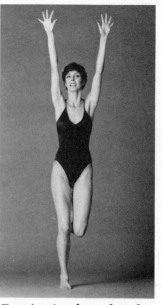

Feet jog in place; hands on your shoulders at shoulder height. Both hands reach up above your head . . .

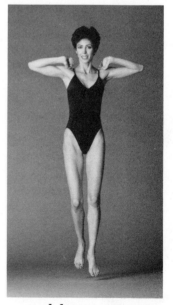

. . . and down to your shoulders in single counts. Keep your shoulders down, moving only your arms.

15
JOGGING
PUNCHES

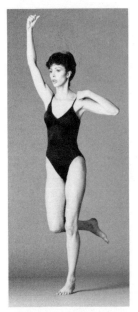

Jog in place; hands on your shoulders. RIGHT hand punches up above your head as LEFT hand remains on LEFT shoulder . . .

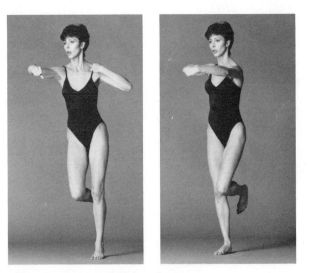

Then, arms punch front from the shoulders, RIGHT and LEFT.

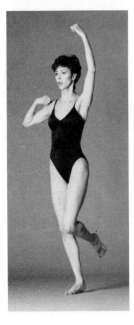

. . . then, LEFT hand punches up above your head as RIGHT hand remains on RIGHT shoulder. Single counts RIGHT and LEFT.

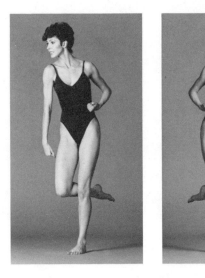

Then, continue to jog and punch hands down toward the floor, RIGHT and LEFT.

16
JOG/ARMS CROSS IN AND OUT

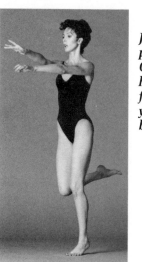

Jog in place. Cross your hands in front of your body . . .

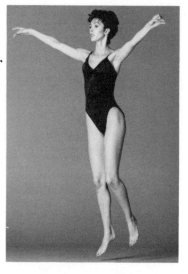

. . . and out at shoulder height. Single counts. Keep your arms straight and tight and your stomach muscles in.

17
JOG/ DIAGONAL ARMS

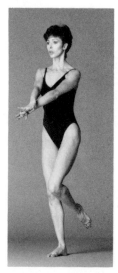

Feet jog in place. Start with your hands crossed low in front of your body.

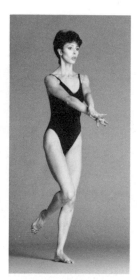

Swing your RIGHT arm diagonally up and back over your head as LEFT arm swings diagonally down and to the back.

Bring hands center.

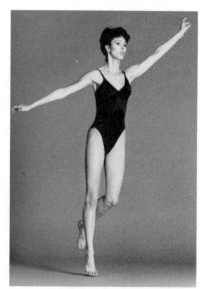

Then, reverse to the other side. LEFT arm swings up and back as RIGHT arm swings down. Up and center make up one count on each side.

18
JOG/STRAIGHT ARM SWINGS

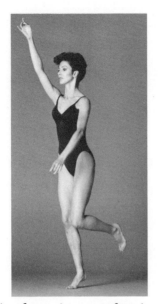

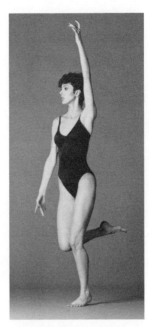

Jog in place. As RIGHT foot is down, RIGHT arm swings straight up above your head.

As LEFT foot is down, LEFT arm swings straight up above your head. Single counts RIGHT and LEFT.

19
STEP KICK

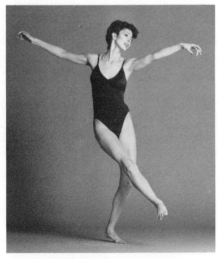

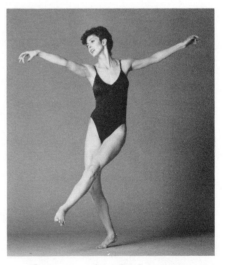

RIGHT foot kicks out front as LEFT arm swings out front at shoulder height and RIGHT arm swings to the back . . .

. . . then, LEFT foot kicks out as RIGHT arm swings front and LEFT arm swings back. This is a nice transitional move. It gives you a chance to take a little breather. Keep it light. It's like walking on air.

20 ELBOW-TO-KNEE LIFTS

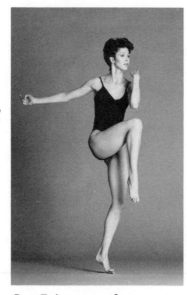
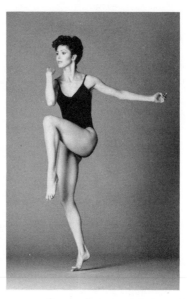

Jog. Bring RIGHT knee up to meet LEFT elbow . . .

. . . and LEFT knee up to meet RIGHT elbow. Single counts.

21 JUMP TOUCH

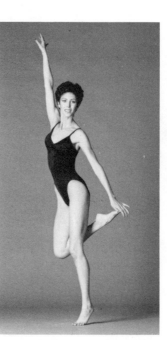
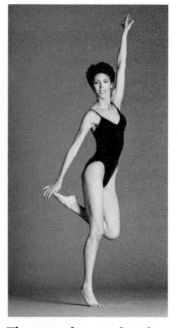

Feet jump together. Then jump on left foot, kicking RIGHT foot back, and touching LEFT hand to RIGHT foot as RIGHT arm swings up straight over head. Jump with feet together.

Then, touch RIGHT hand to LEFT foot as LEFT arm swings up straight.

22 Cross Jumps

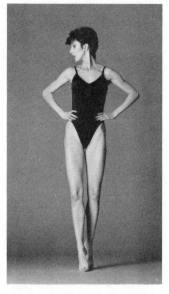 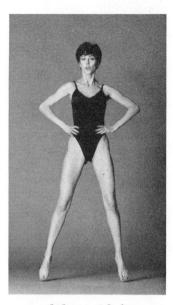

With your hands on your waist, jump, crossing your feet at the ankles . . .

. . . and then with feet out at shoulder width. Alternate crossing RIGHT and then LEFT foot in front. Keep your legs straight and your stomach muscles held in.

23 Half-Jacks

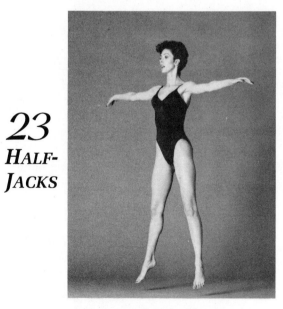 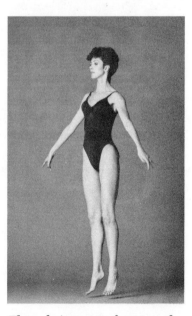

Jump up and out with your legs, landing on the balls of your feet, as arms swing up to shoulder height.

Then, bring your feet together as arms come down to your sides. Up and down make up one count.

24 JUMPING JACKS

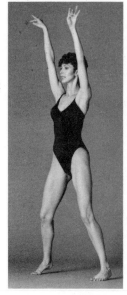

Jump up and out with your legs, landing on the balls of your feet as your arms swing up freely from the shoulders above your head.

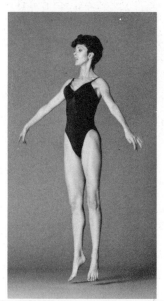

Then, bring your feet together as arms come down to your sides. Up and down make up one count.

25 HEEL JACKS

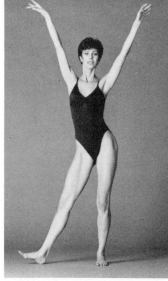

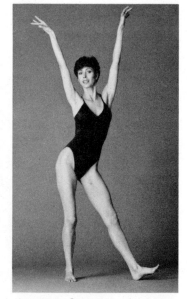

As you hop and land on LEFT foot, RIGHT foot points with toes upward. LEFT hip thrusts forward and arms swing up above your head.

Come to center briefly.

Reverse, hopping on RIGHT foot, pointing LEFT toes upward, thrusting RIGHT hip forward and swinging arms above your head.

26
AEROBIC SIDE LUNGE

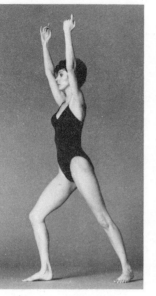 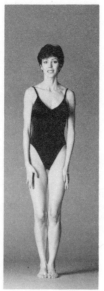 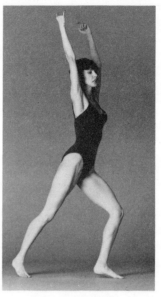

Start with feet more than shoulder width apart. Lunge body to the RIGHT, bending RIGHT leg. LEFT leg is straight. Both arms swing up above your head to the RIGHT.

Jump center.

Then lunge LEFT, bending LEFT leg while RIGHT leg is straight, and swing both arms up to the LEFT. You should feel the stretch throughout your body, from your calves through your upper arms. Keep it fluid as you lunge side to side by using your arms for momentum.

27
ONE- ARM LUNGE

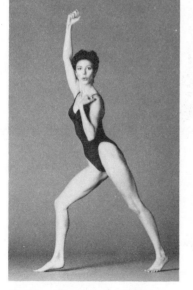 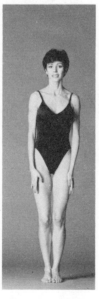 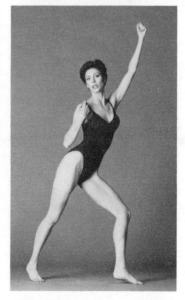

Start with feet more than shoulder width apart. Lunge body and RIGHT leg to the RIGHT. RIGHT arm swings up straight as LEFT arm is bent into your body.

Jump center.

Then, lunge LEFT with LEFT leg bent. LEFT arm swings up straight. Again, feel the stretch all through your body.

28
TWISTS

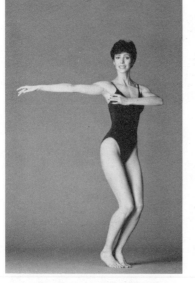 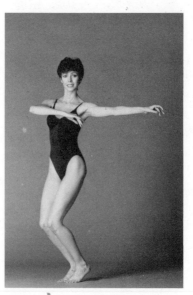

Jump with feet together and knees bent, twisting to the LEFT as arms cross the body at shoulder height to the RIGHT.

Then, twist to the RIGHT as arms cross the body at shoulder height to the LEFT. Two counts on each side. Then, single twists.

29
ARM MEETS THE LEG

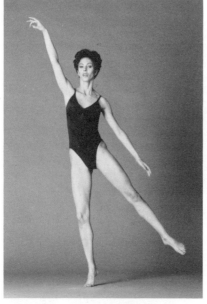 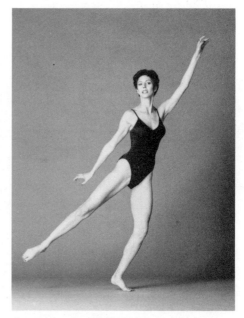

Hop on one foot as you swing other leg out to side; feet move side to side. As RIGHT arm swings up straight from the shoulder, LEFT arm is down at your side to meet extended LEFT leg.

As LEFT arm swings up, RIGHT arm meets extended RIGHT leg. Single counts.

30
HAND TO HEEL

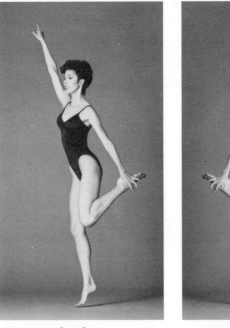
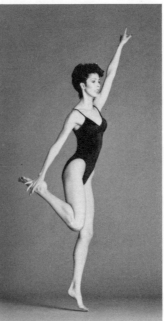

Jog. LEFT heel comes up to meet LEFT hand . . .

. . . then RIGHT heel comes up to meet RIGHT hand. Single counts LEFT and RIGHT.

31
WILD JUMPS

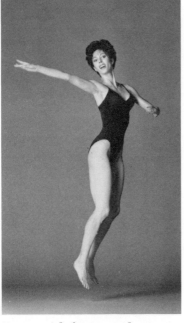
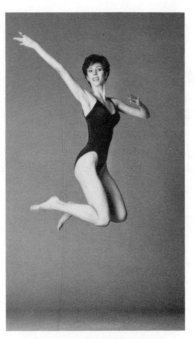

Jump with feet together . . .

. . . then jump and bring heels up and close to buttocks. This is an advanced move and will take some patience. Have fun with it. Be wild!

32
JOG/HANDS CROSS LOW

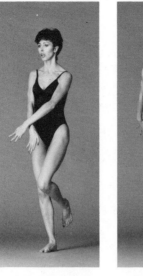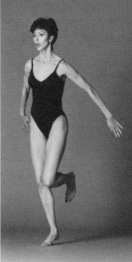

Jog. Hands cross low in front of body 4 counts . . .

. . . and low behind 4 counts. Then single counts front and back.

33
JOG/ARM RELEASE

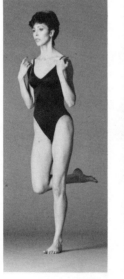

Slowly jog in place as lower arms bend in to chest . . .

. . . and down straight to the back.

10
JOG

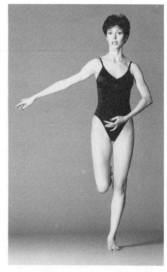

Slowly jog in place, cooling it down. You must cool down after aerobics to bring your heart rate back to its resting state.

5
TWO-ARM STANDING LUNGE

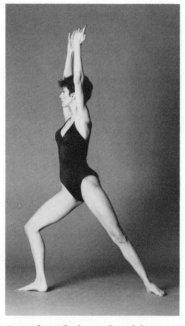 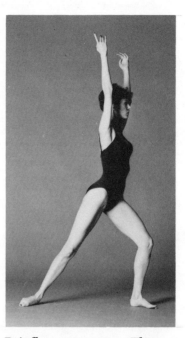

Stand with feet shoulder width apart; arms at your side. Slowly lunge body and RIGHT leg to the RIGHT for 2 counts as both arms swing up above your head.

Briefly come center. Then lunge body and LEFT leg to the LEFT for 2 counts. This is a great overall stretch after aerobics. Keep it fluid, allowing your body to cool down gradually.

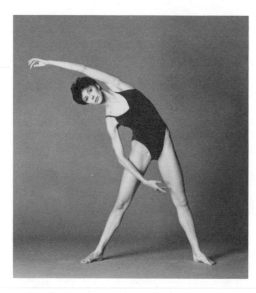

34
FLAT-BACK FOLLOW-THROUGH

Stand with feet more than shoulder width apart; stomach muscles in; hips tucked under. LEFT arm reaches over to the RIGHT, getting a good stretch in the LEFT side; RIGHT arm curves low in front of body; hold 4 counts.

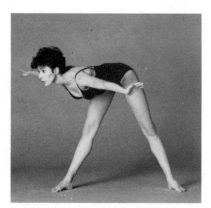

Bend with a flat back over to the RIGHT; arms out at shoulder level parallel to the floor; hold 4 counts.

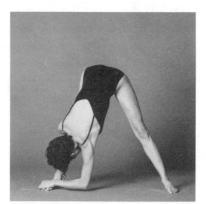

Drop your head to your RIGHT knee and hold your ankles with your hands; 4 counts. Feel the stretch in the back of your legs.

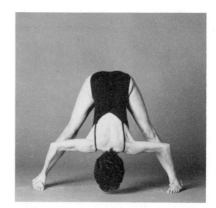

Come center with a flat back; hold hands on ankles; 4 counts. Pull out from the spine.

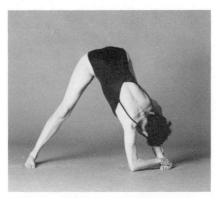

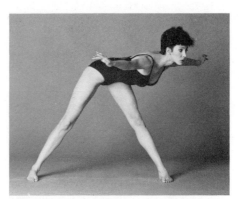

Drop your head to your LEFT knee; hands to ankles; hold 4 counts.

Flat back to the LEFT; arms out at shoulder level parallel to the floor; 4 counts.

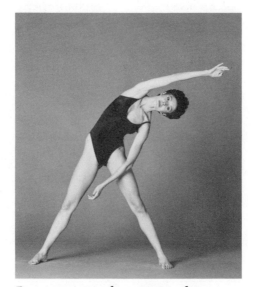

RIGHT arm reaches over to the LEFT; LEFT arm curves low in front of your body; 4 counts.

35
PUPPET

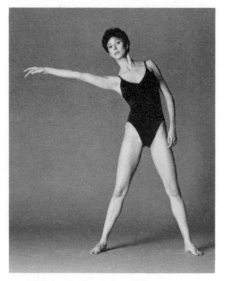
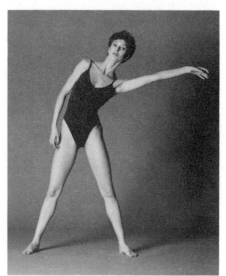

Stand with feet shoulder width apart; arms down at your sides. RIGHT arm reaches out at shoulder height as if pulled on a string. Feel the stretch in your LEFT side.

Then, LEFT arm reaches out at shoulder height. Feel the stretch in the RIGHT side. Keep your stomach muscles held in and your body front.

36
SHOULDER LEADS

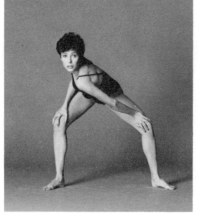
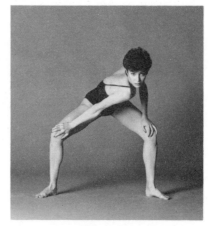

Stand with feet wide apart; legs bent; hands on your knees. Twist your torso and press your LEFT shoulder front 2 counts, feeling the stretch in your LEFT side.

Then, twist your torso and press your RIGHT shoulder front 2 counts, feeling the stretch in your RIGHT side.

37
HEEL
RAISES
& PRESSES

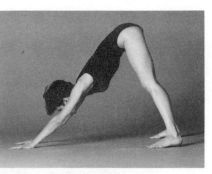

Start with feet wide apart behind; arms out straight with hands apart on the floor in front of you; your legs are straight; back is flat.

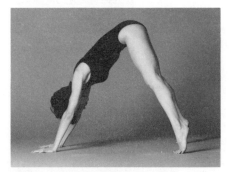

Raise up and down on your toes, in single counts, stretching your calves.

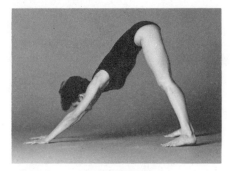

Then, press your heels down and your chest toward the floor. Hold for 4 counts.

38
TENDON STRETCH

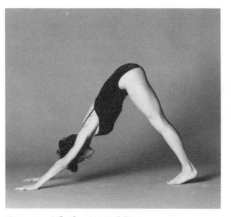

Start with feet and legs together and straight behind; arms out straight with hands apart on the floor in front of you.

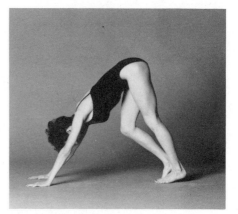

Raise RIGHT heel up, bending RIGHT knee as you press LEFT heel to the floor for 2 counts.

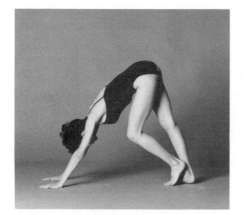

Raise LEFT heel up, bending LEFT knee as you press RIGHT heel to the floor for 2 counts, then single counts.

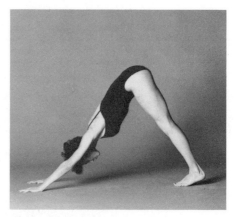

Then, press your heels to the floor and hold the stretch.

39
SHOULDER STAND
TO PLOUGH

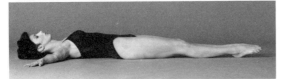

Lie on your back.

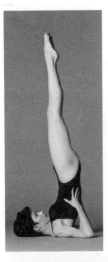

Swing your feet up straight in the air, supporting your back with your hands. This allows the blood to flow back to your brain after aerobics. Hold this position for 15 seconds.

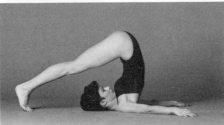

Then, extend your legs straight out behind you. Arms may be out to the side or on your back for support. Hold for 30 seconds.

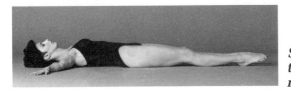

40
REACH
OVER

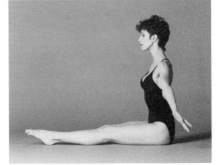

Sit up, arms out at shoulder height, stomach held in.

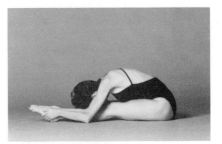

With a flat back, reach over toward ankles as far as you can, bringing your head to your knees. Hold for a count of 10.

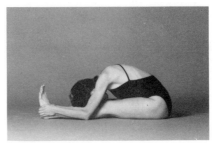

Point and flex your feet.

Slowly roll your legs down to the floor in front of you and relax.

Chapter Five

The Aerobicise WORKOUTS

The workouts are divided into three sections—Warm-Up, Aerobics, and Cool-Down. The Warm-up prepares your muscular and skeletal systems. Cold muscles can be easily injured. Therefore, it is absolutely necessary to warm up before you move on to the more strenuous cardiovascular activities.

Warming up your body encourages the acceleration of your heart rate. And by increasing your heart rate, your blood can more easily carry the oxygen through your tissues, thereby nourishing and stimulating them.

Aerobics are those activities that improve your cardiovascular fitness. Our aerobic routines are laid out in such a way that you can begin gradually and work your way up to 12 continuous minutes a day. For most people, the aerobic part of the workout is the most enjoyable. It's fast, fun, and will leave you feeling full of life.

Like the Warm-up, the Cool-Down is an essential part of your workout. It helps your heart rate, blood pressure, and body temperature return to their preexercise levels. It will also ease aching muscles by stretching out those areas you used in the aerobic section. If you do nothing else after aerobics, at least walk around for a few minutes to help your heart rate return to normal.

THREE MINUTES TO BEGIN · IF YOU ARE VERY OUT OF SHAPE

WARM-UP · ONE MINUTE
(Music—96 Beats Per Minute)

1

**HEAD
TILTS
AND TURNS**
(30 SECONDS)

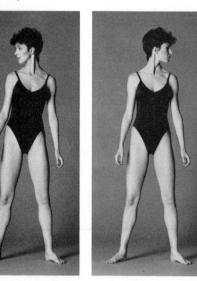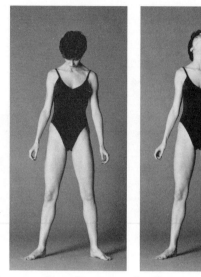

Stand; feet shoulder width apart; stomach held in; hips tucked under; arms at your sides. Head looks RIGHT and LEFT . . .

. . . then front and back.

2

**RIB
ISOLATION**
(30 SECONDS)

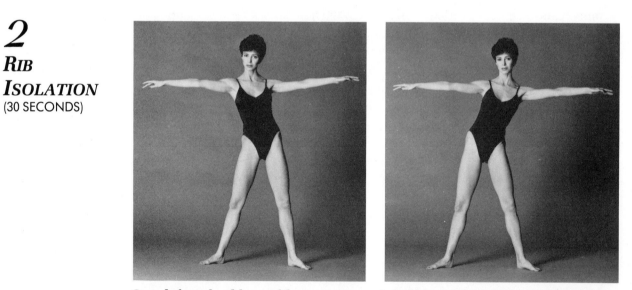

Stand; feet shoulder width apart; stomach held in; hips tucked under; arms out at shoulder height. Concentrate on moving just your rib cage RIGHT and LEFT. Keep your shoulders down.

AEROBICS · ONE MINUTE
(Music—108 Beats Per Minute)

10
JOG
(30 SECONDS)

Pick your feet up lightly. Land on the balls of your feet and work it through the heels. Keep it light.

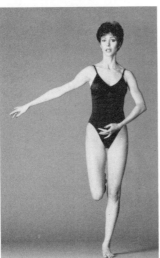

11
JOG/ARM CIRCLES
(30 SECONDS)

Feet jog in place. Arms out at shoulder height. Circle arms front with palms down 4 counts. Circle back with palms up 4 counts.

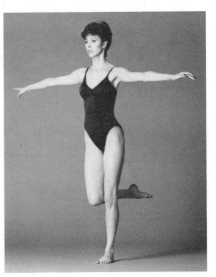

COOL-DOWN · 1 MINUTE
(Music—96 Beats Per Minute)

5
TWO-ARM STANDING LUNGE
(30 SECONDS)

Stand with feet shoulder width apart; arms at your sides. Slowly lunge body and RIGHT leg to the RIGHT 2 counts as both arms swing up above your head, then LEFT 2 counts, cooling it down.

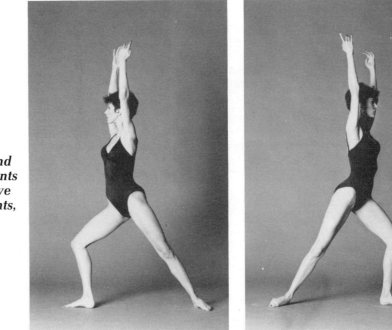

34
FLAT-BACK FOLLOW-THROUGH
(30 SECONDS)

Feet apart; LEFT arm reaches over to the RIGHT as RIGHT arm curves low in front of body; hold 4 counts. Flat back to the RIGHT; arms out at shoulder level; 4 counts. Drop head to RIGHT knee; hands to ankle; 4 counts. Come center; hands to ankles; 4 counts. Head to LEFT knee; hands to ankles; 4 counts. Flat back to the LEFT; arms out at shoulder level; 4 counts. RIGHT arm reaches over to the LEFT as LEFT arm curves low in front of body; 4 counts.

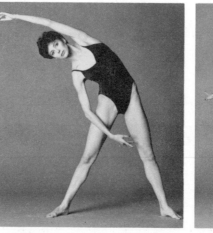
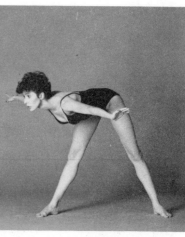

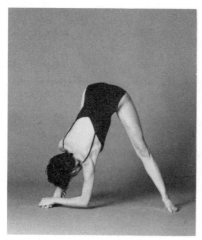
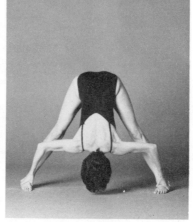
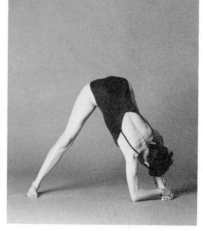

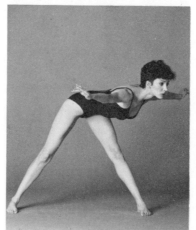
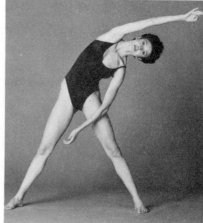

Warm-Up · 2 Minutes
(Music—102 Beats Per Minute)

1

HEAD TILTS AND TURNS
(30 SECONDS)

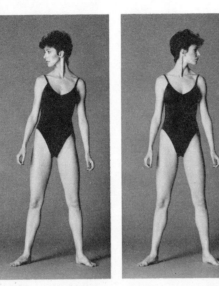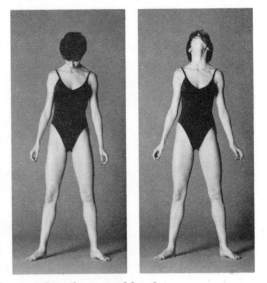

Stand; feet shoulder width apart; stomach held in; hips tucked under; arms at your sides. Head looks RIGHT and LEFT . . .   *. . . then front and back.*

2

RIB ISOLATION
(30 SECONDS)

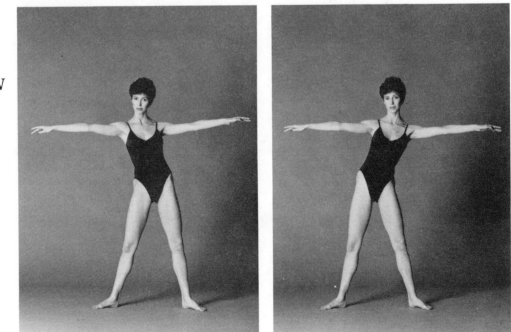

Stand; feet shoulder width apart; stomach held in; hips tucked under; arms out at shoulder height. Concentrate on moving just your rib cage RIGHT and LEFT. Keep your shoulders down.

3
SIDE STRETCHES
(30 SECONDS)

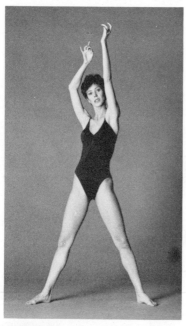
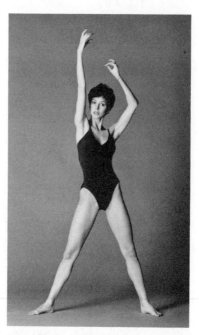

Stand; feet shoulder width apart. Reach up with your LEFT arm 2 counts, feeling the stretch in your LEFT side.

Reach up with your RIGHT arm 2 counts. Stretch up and out from the rib cage. Then, single counts LEFT and RIGHT.

4
BOW & ARROW
(30 SECONDS)

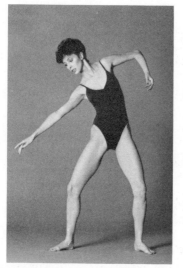
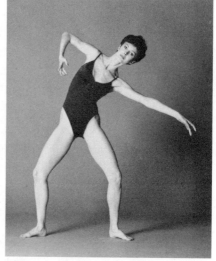

Stand with feet shoulder width apart; knees slightly bent. Starting to the RIGHT, reach RIGHT arm out straight as LEFT arm bows up. Feel the stretch in your LEFT side. Come back to center.

Reverse to the LEFT. Be sure to pull directly to the side, keeping your body front. Single counts RIGHT and LEFT.

AEROBICS · THREE MINUTES
(Music—114 Beats Per Minute)

10
JOG
(30 SECONDS)

Pick up your feet lightly. Land on the balls of your feet and work it through the heels. Keep it light.

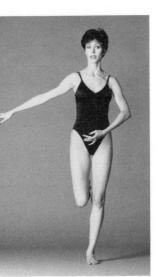

11
JOG/ARM CIRCLES
(30 SECONDS)

Feet jog in place. Arms out at shoulder height. Circle arms front with palms down 4 counts. Circle back with palms up 4 counts.

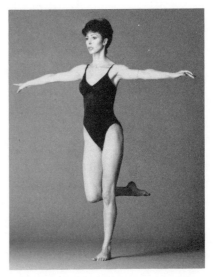

12
JOG/PUSH FRONT
(30 SECONDS)

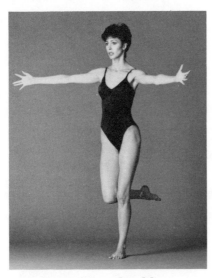

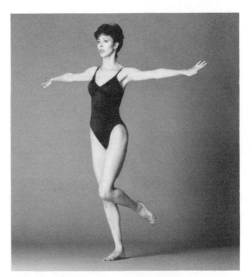

Jog. Arms out at shoulder height. Arms push front with palms front 4 counts.

Then, arms push back with palms back 4 counts.

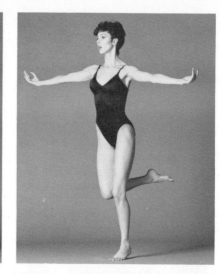

13
JOG/HANDS TO SHOULDERS
(30 SECONDS)

Jog. Arms out at shoulder height. Keep your upper arms still as you bring hands to shoulders and back out straight.

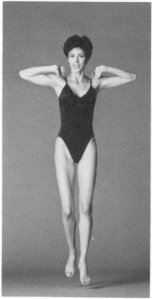

14
JOG/ REACH UP
(30 SECONDS)

Continue jogging. Both hands reach up above your head and down to your shoulders.

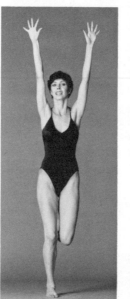

15 JOGGING PUNCHES (30 SECONDS)

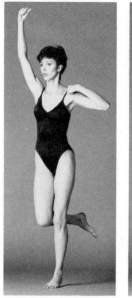
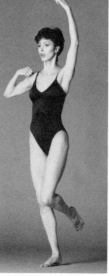
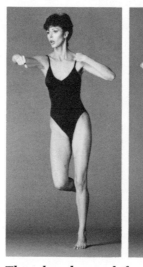
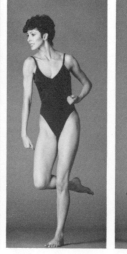

Jog in place. Hands punch up from the shoulders RIGHT and LEFT.

Then, hands punch front RIGHT and LEFT.

Then, continue to jog and punch hands down toward the floor RIGHT and LEFT.

COOL-DOWN · ONE MINUTE
(Music—102 Beats Per Minute)

5

TWO-ARM STANDING LUNGE (30 SECONDS)

Stand with feet shoulder width apart; arms at your sides. Slowly lunge body and RIGHT leg RIGHT. 2 counts as both arms swing up above your head, then LEFT 2 counts, cooling it down.

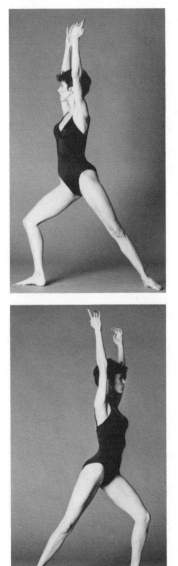

34 FLAT-BACK FOLLOW- THROUGH
(30 SECONDS)

Feet apart; LEFT arm reaches over to the RIGHT as RIGHT arm curves low in front of body; hold 4 counts. Flat back to the RIGHT; arms out at shoulder level; 4 counts. Drop head to RIGHT knee; hands to ankle; 4 counts. Come center; hands to ankles; 4 counts. Head to LEFT knee; hands to ankles; 4 counts. Flat back to the LEFT; arms out at shoulder level; 4 counts. RIGHT arm reaches over to the LEFT as LEFT arm curves low in front of body; 4 counts.

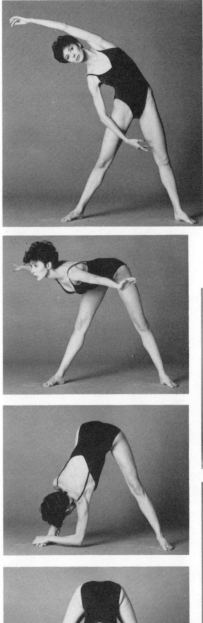

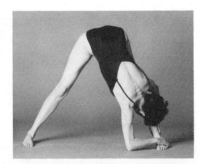

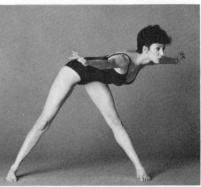

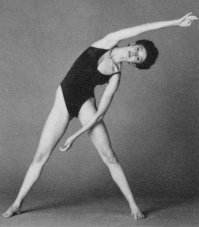

WARM-UP · 2 MINUTES
(Music—108 Beats Per Minute)

3

SIDE STRETCHES
(30 SECONDS)

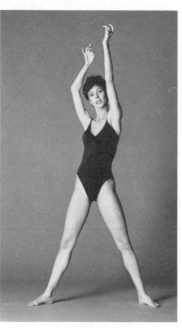 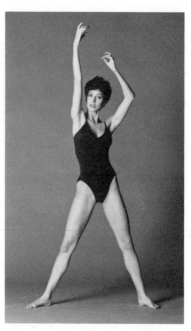

Stand; feet shoulder width apart. Reach up with your LEFT arm 2 counts, feeling the stretch in your LEFT side.

Reach up with your RIGHT arm 2 counts. Stretch up and out from the rib cage. Then, single counts LEFT and RIGHT.

4

BOW & ARROW
(30 SECONDS)

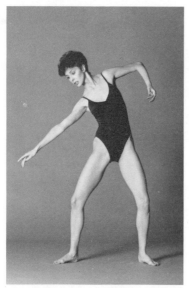 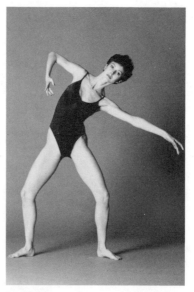

Stand with feet shoulder width apart; knees slightly bent. Starting to the RIGHT, reach RIGHT arm out straight as LEFT arm bows up. Feel the stretch in your LEFT side. Come back to center.

Reverse to the LEFT. Be sure to pull directly to the side, keeping your body front. Single counts RIGHT and LEFT.

5
TWO-ARM STANDING LUNGE
(30 SECONDS)

Feet wide apart; arms at sides; lunge body and RIGHT leg to the RIGHT as both arms swing up above head to the RIGHT. Come center. Then, lunge LEFT. Keep it fluid. Use your arms for momentum.

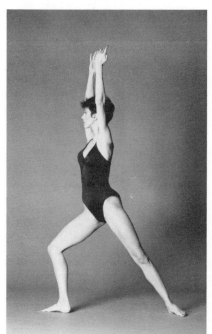 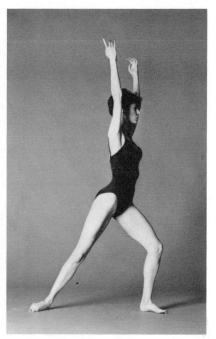

6
ELBOW-TO-KNEE LUNGE
(30 SECONDS)

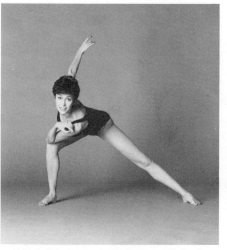 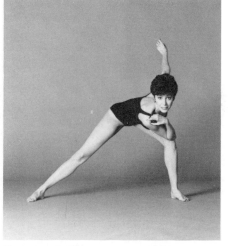

With a flat back, lunge to the RIGHT, reaching LEFT elbow to RIGHT knee and letting your RIGHT arm swing up toward the ceiling.

Reverse to the LEFT, reaching RIGHT elbow to LEFT knee in single counts.

AEROBICS · 5 MINUTES
(Music—120 Beats Per Minute)

10
JOG
(30 SECONDS)

Pick up your feet lightly. Land on the balls of your feet and work it through the heels. Keep it light.

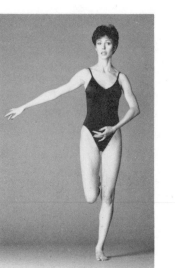

11
JOG/ARM CIRCLES
(30 SECONDS)

Feet jog in place. Arms out at shoulder height. Circle arms front with palms down 4 counts. Circle back with palms up 4 counts.

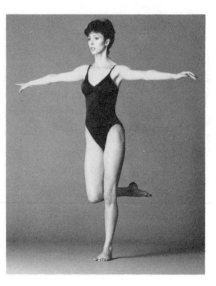

12
JOG/PUSH FRONT
(30 SECONDS)

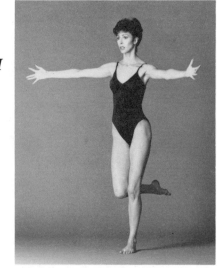

Jog. Arms out at shoulder height. Arms push front with palms front 4 counts.

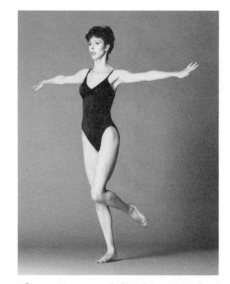

Then, arms push back with palms back 4 counts.

13
JOG/HANDS TO SHOULDERS
(30 SECONDS)

Jog. Arms out at shoulder height. Keep your upper arms still as you bring hands to shoulders and back out straight.

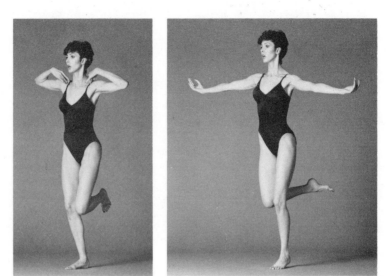

14
JOG/ REACH UP
(30 SECONDS)

Continue jogging. Both hands reach up above your head and down to your shoulders.

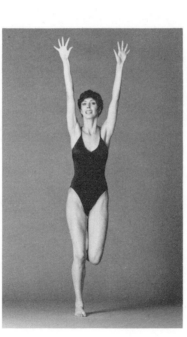
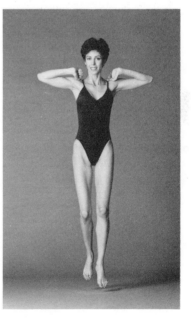

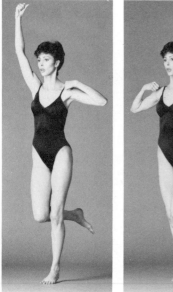
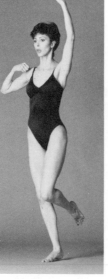

15 JOGGING PUNCHES (30 SECONDS)

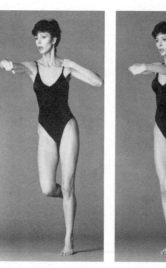
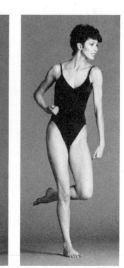

Jog in place. Hands punch up from the shoulders **RIGHT** and **LEFT**.

Then, hands punch front **RIGHT** and **LEFT**.

Then, continue to jog and punch hands down toward the floor **RIGHT** and **LEFT**.

16
JOG/ARMS CROSS IN AND OUT
(30 SECONDS)

Jog in place. Cross your hands in front of your body and out at shoulder height. Single counts.

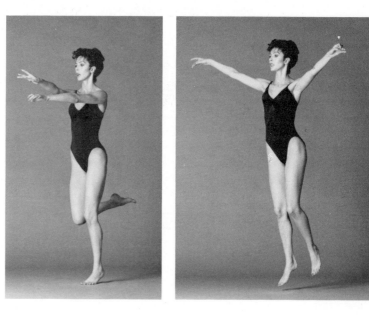

17
JOG/ DIAGONAL ARMS
(30 SECONDS)

Feet jog in place. Cross your hands low in front of your body, then up and out diagonally, alternating RIGHT and LEFT.

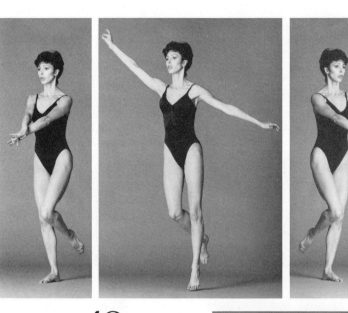

18
JOG/ STRAIGHT ARM SWINGS
(30 SECONDS)

Continue jogging. As RIGHT heel is down, RIGHT arm swings up. Then, as LEFT heel is down, LEFT arm swings up.

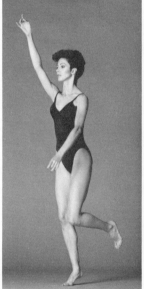
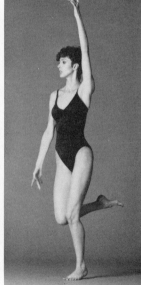

19
STEP KICK
(30 SECONDS)

RIGHT foot kicks out front as LEFT arm swings out front and RIGHT arm swings back. Then, LEFT foot kicks out as RIGHT arm swings front and LEFT arm swings back.

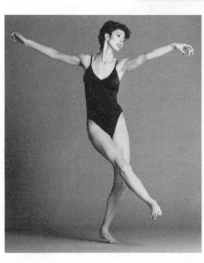
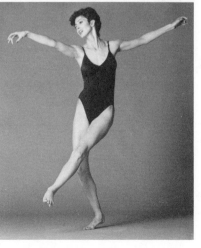

COOL-DOWN · 2 MINUTES
(Music—108 Beats Per Minute)

5
TWO-ARM STANDING LUNGE
(30 SECONDS)

Stand with feet shoulder width apart; arms at your sides. Slowly lunge body RIGHT 2 counts and LEFT 2 counts, cooling it down.

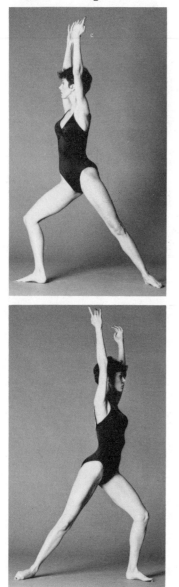

34 FLAT-BACK FOLLOW-THROUGH
(30 SECONDS)

Feet apart; LEFT arm reaches over to the RIGHT as RIGHT arm curves low in front of body; hold 4 counts. Flat back to the RIGHT; arms out at shoulder level; 4 counts. Drop head to RIGHT knee; hands to ankle; 4 counts. Come center; hands to ankles; 4 counts.

Head to LEFT knee; hands to ankles; 4 counts. Flat back to the LEFT; arms out at shoulder level; 4 counts. RIGHT arm reaches over to the LEFT as LEFT arm curves low in front of body; 4 counts.

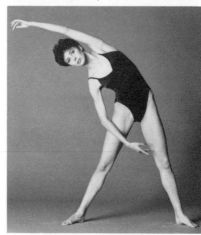

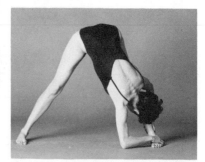

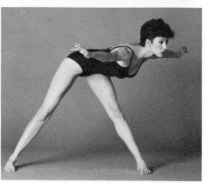

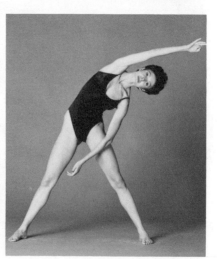

35
PUPPET
(30 SECONDS)

*Feet shoulder width apart;
arms at your sides. RIGHT arm
reaches out at shoulder
height as if pulled on a string.
Reverse to the LEFT.*

36
SHOULDER
LEADS
(30 SECONDS)

*Feet wide apart; legs bent;
hands on knees. Twist your
torso and press LEFT shoulder
front 2 counts, then RIGHT
shoulder front 2 counts.*

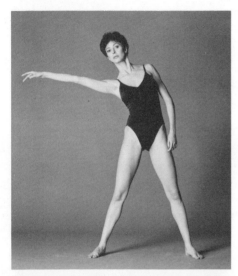

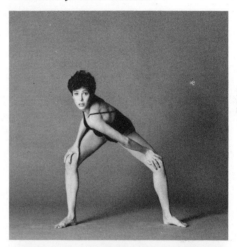

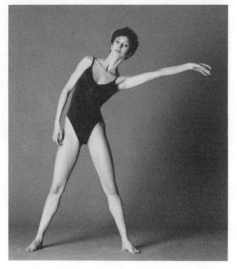

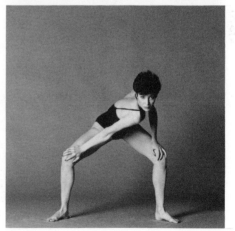

12 Minutes for Life · If You Are in Shape

Warm-Up · 2 Minutes
(Music—114 Beats Per Minute)

3

**Side
Stretches**
(30 SECONDS)

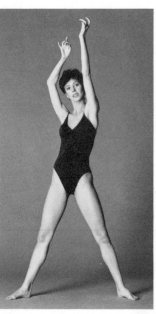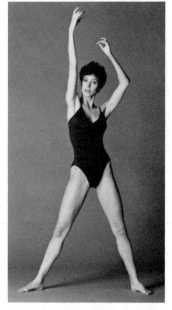

Stand; feet shoulder width apart. Reach up with your LEFT arm 2 counts, feeling the stretch in your LEFT side.

Reach up with your RIGHT arm 2 counts. Stretch up and out from the rib cage. Then, single counts LEFT and RIGHT.

4

**Bow &
Arrow**
(30 SECONDS)

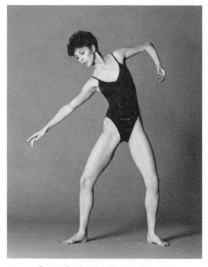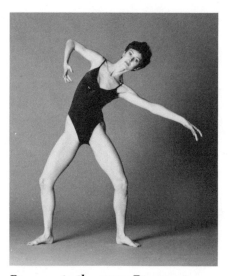

Stand with feet shoulder width apart; knees slightly bent. Starting to the RIGHT, reach RIGHT arm out straight as LEFT arm bows up. Feel the stretch in your LEFT side. Come back to center.

Reverse to the LEFT. Be sure to pull directly to the side, keeping your body front. Single counts RIGHT and LEFT.

5
TWO-ARM STANDING LUNGE
(30 SECONDS)

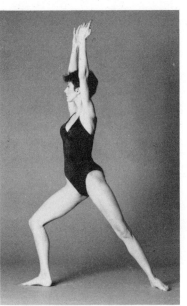 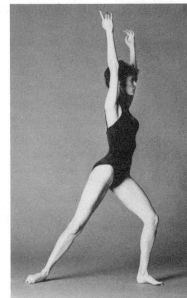

Feet wide apart; arms at sides. Lunge body and RIGHT leg to the RIGHT as both arms swing up above head to the RIGHT. Come center.

Then, lunge LEFT. Keep it fluid. Use your arms for momentum.

6
ELBOW-TO-KNEE LUNGE
(30 SECONDS)

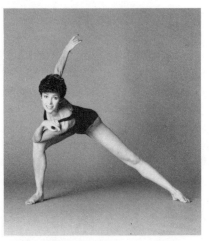 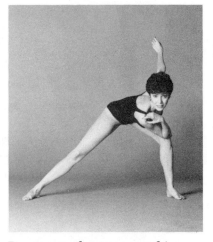

With a flat back, lunge to the RIGHT, reaching LEFT elbow to RIGHT knee and letting your RIGHT arm swing up toward the ceiling.

Reverse to the LEFT, reaching RIGHT elbow to LEFT knee in single counts.

10
JOG
(30 SECONDS)

Pick up your feet lightly.
Land on the balls of your feet
and work it through the heels.
Keep it light.

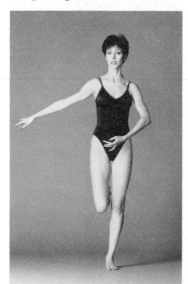

11
JOG/ARM
CIRCLES
(30 SECONDS)

Feet jog in place. Arms out at
shoulder height. Circle arms
front with palms down 4 counts.
Circle back with palms up 4 counts.

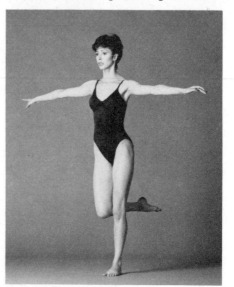

12
JOG/PUSH
FRONT
(30 SECONDS)

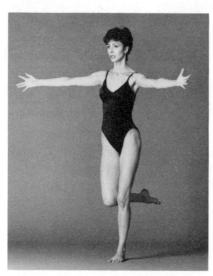

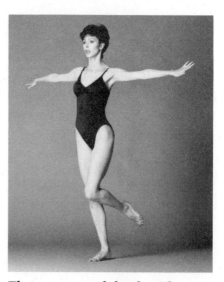

Jog. Arms out at shoulder
height. Arms push front with
palms front 4 counts.

Then, arms push back with
palms back 4 counts.

13

JOG/HANDS TO SHOULDERS
(30 SECONDS)

Jog. Arms out at shoulder height. Keep your upper arms still as you bring hands to shoulders and back out straight.

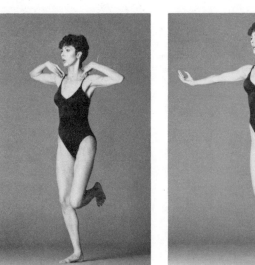
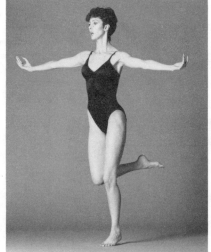

14

JOG/ REACH UP
(30 SECONDS)

Continue jogging. Both hands reach up above your head and down to your shoulders.

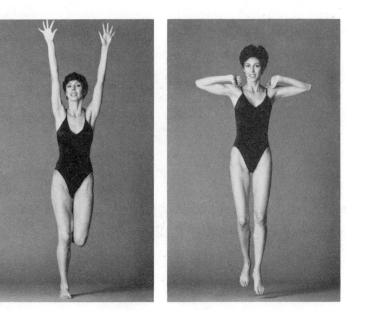

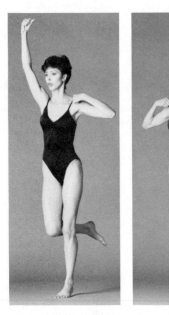

15 JOGGING PUNCHES (30 SECONDS)

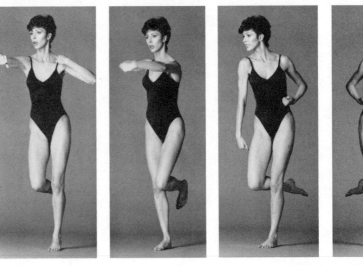

Jog in place. Hands punch up from the shoulders RIGHT and LEFT.

Then, hands punch front RIGHT and LEFT.

Then, continue to jog and punch hands down toward the floor RIGHT and LEFT.

16 JOG/ARMS CROSS IN AND OUT (30 SECONDS)

Jog in place. Cross your hands in front of your body and out at shoulder height. Single counts.

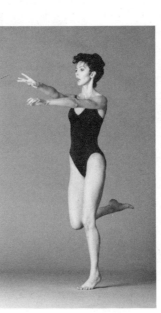

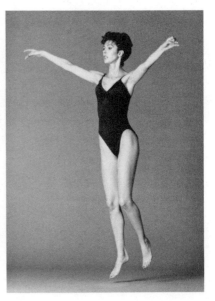

17
JOG/ DIAGONAL ARMS
(30 SECONDS)

Feet jog in place. Cross your hands low in front of your body, then up and out diagonally, alternating RIGHT *and* LEFT.

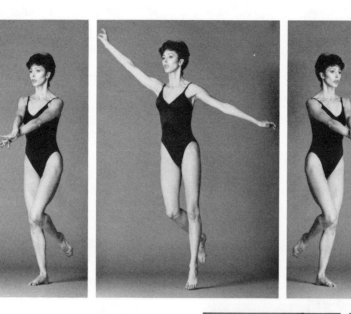
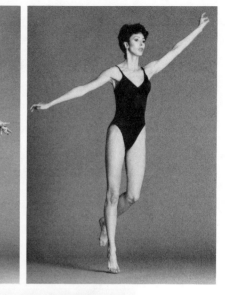

18
JOG/ STRAIGHT ARM SWINGS
(30 SECONDS)

Continue jogging. As RIGHT *heel is down,* RIGHT *arm swings up. Then, as* LEFT *heel is down,* LEFT *arm swings up.*

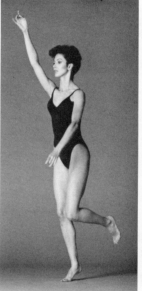
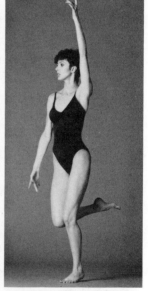

19
STEP KICK
(30 SECONDS)

RIGHT foot kicks out front as LEFT arm swings out front and RIGHT arm swings back. Then, LEFT foot kicks out as RIGHT arm swings front and LEFT arm swings back.

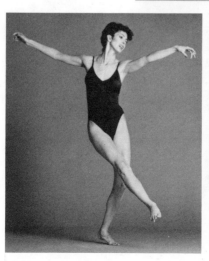
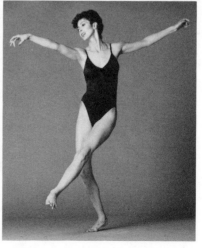

20
ELBOW-TO-
KNEE
LIFTS
(30 SECONDS)

Jog. Bring RIGHT knee up to meet LEFT elbow. Reverse, LEFT knee comes up to meet RIGHT elbow.

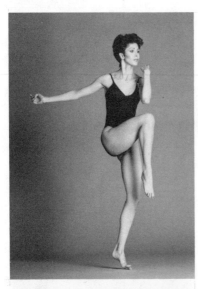

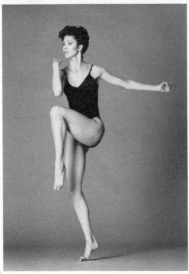

21
JUMP
TOUCH
(30 SECONDS)

Feet jump together. Then alternate touching LEFT hand to RIGHT foot and RIGHT hand to LEFT foot in back of you, with free arm swinging over head.

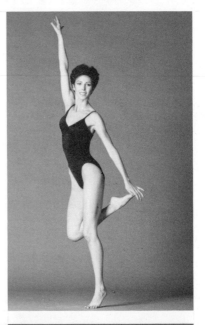

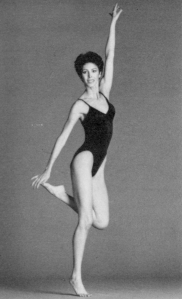

22
CROSS
JUMPS
(30 SECONDS)

Hands on waist. Jump. Feet cross at ankles and then out shoulder width. Alternate, crossing RIGHT then LEFT foot in front.

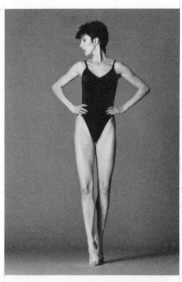

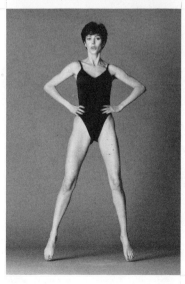

23
HALF-
JACKS
(30 SECONDS)

Jump up and out with your feet as arms swing up to shoulder height. Then, bring your feet together as arms come down to your sides.

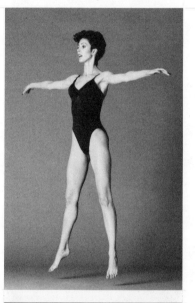

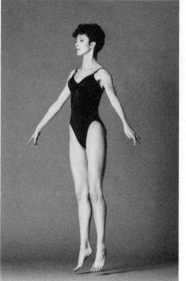

24
JUMPING JACKS
(30 SECONDS)

Jump up and out with your feet as your arms swing up freely from the shoulders above your head. Then, bring your feet together as arms come down.

25
HEEL JACKS
(30 SECONDS)

As you hop on LEFT foot, extend RIGHT foot out to side and touch RIGHT heel to floor, toes pointed upward. Thrust hip outward and swing arms above head. Alternate.

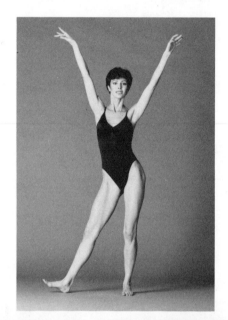

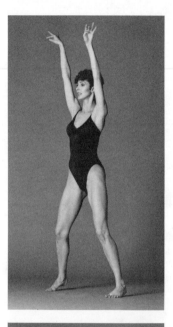

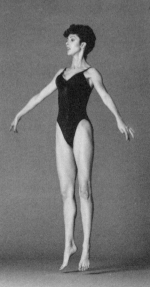

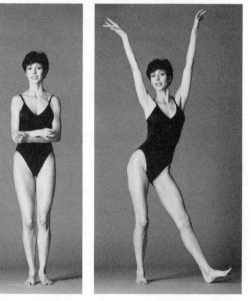

COOL-DOWN · 2 MINUTES
(Music—114 Beats Per Minute)

5
TWO-ARM STANDING LUNGE
(30 SECONDS)

Stand with feet shoulder width apart; arms at your sides. Slowly lunge body RIGHT 2 counts and LEFT 2 counts, cooling it down.

36
SHOULDER LEADS
(30 SECONDS)

Feet wide apart; legs bent; hands on knees. Twist your torso and press LEFT shoulder front 2 counts, then RIGHT shoulder front 2 counts.

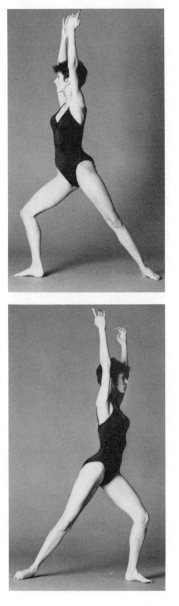

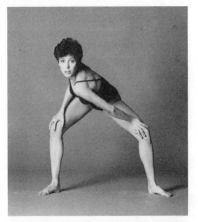

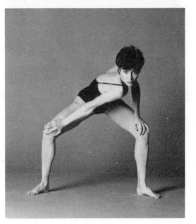

37
HEEL RAISES
& PRESSES
(30 SECONDS)

Feet wide apart behind; hands apart on the floor in front of you; legs straight; back flat. Raise up and down on your toes in single counts, stretching your calves. Then, press your heels down and your chest toward the floor and hold 4 counts.

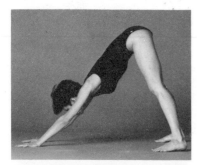

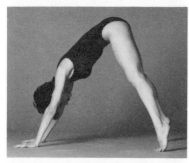

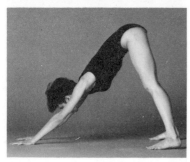

38
TENDON
STRETCH
(30 SECONDS)

Start with hands on the floor and feet and legs together and behind. Raise RIGHT heel up, bending RIGHT knee as you press LEFT heel to the floor for 2 counts. Reverse for the LEFT heel. Then, single counts. Then, heels to the floor and hold the stretch.

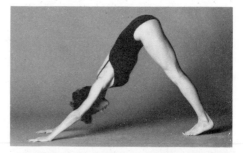

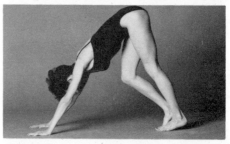

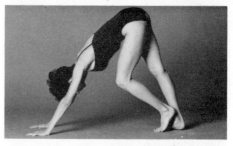

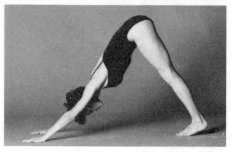

WARM-UP · 3 MINUTES
(Music—120 Beats Per Minute)

3

SIDE STRETCHES
(30 SECONDS)

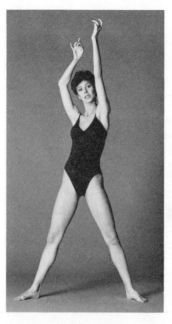 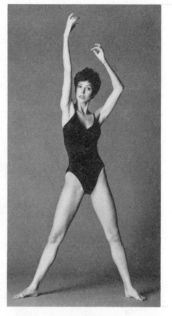

Stand; feet shoulder width apart. Reach up with your LEFT arm 2 counts, feeling the stretch in your LEFT side.

Reach up with your RIGHT arm 2 counts. Stretch up and out from the rib cage. Then, single counts LEFT and RIGHT.

4

BOW & ARROW
(30 SECONDS)

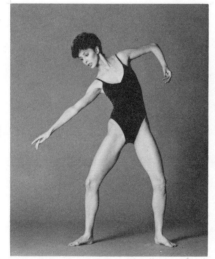 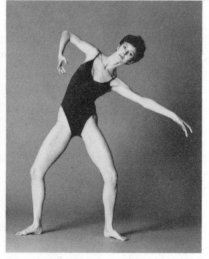

Stand with feet shoulder width apart; knees slightly bent. Starting to the RIGHT, reach RIGHT arm out straight as LEFT arm bows up. Feel the stretch in your LEFT side. Come back to center.

Reverse to the LEFT. Be sure to pull directly to the side, keeping your body front. Single counts RIGHT and LEFT.

5
TWO-ARM STANDING LUNGE
(30 SECONDS)

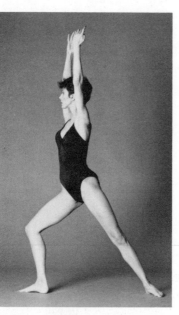
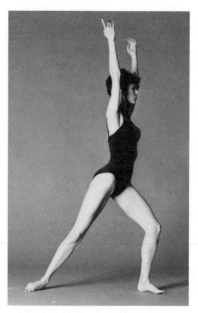

Feet wide apart; arms at sides; lunge body and RIGHT leg to the RIGHT as both arms swing up above head to the RIGHT. Come center.

Then, lunge LEFT. Keep it fluid. Use your arms for momentum.

6
ELBOW-TO-KNEE LUNGE
(30 SECONDS)

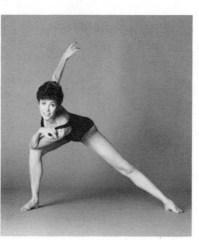
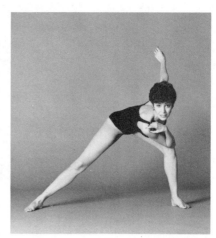

With a flat back, lunge to the RIGHT, reaching LEFT elbow to RIGHT knee and let your RIGHT arm swing up toward the ceiling.

Reverse to the LEFT, reaching RIGHT elbow to LEFT knee in single counts.

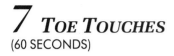

7 TOE TOUCHES
(60 SECONDS)

Continue lunging, but reach LEFT elbow to the floor. Reverse with the RIGHT elbow. Reach down as far as you can. Keep your back flat.

With straight legs, alternate reaching LEFT hand to RIGHT foot and RIGHT hand to LEFT foot. Let your other arm swing up behind you. Single counts.

Now, reach LEFT hand behind RIGHT foot and RIGHT hand behind LEFT foot in single counts.

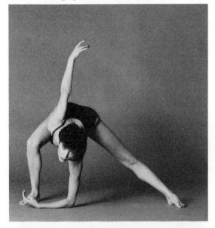

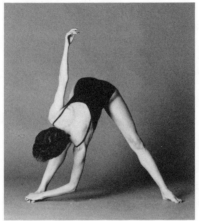

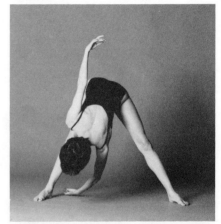

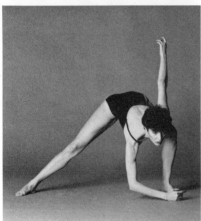

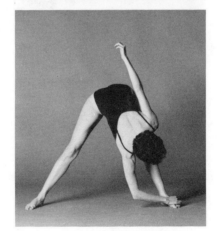

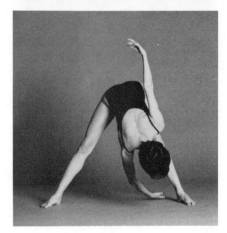

10
JOG
(30 SECONDS)

Pick up your feet lightly. Land on the balls of your feet and work it through the heels. Keep it light.

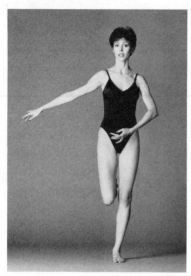

11
JOG/ARM CIRCLES
(30 SECONDS)

Feet jog in place. Arms out at shoulder height. Circle arms front with palms down 4 counts. Circle back with palms up 4 counts.

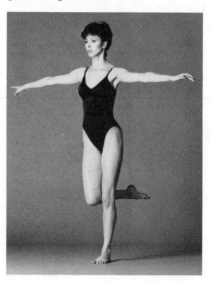

12
JOG/PUSH FRONT
(30 SECONDS)

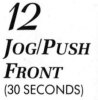

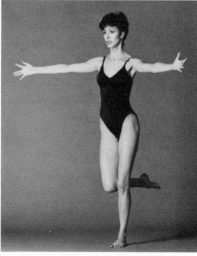

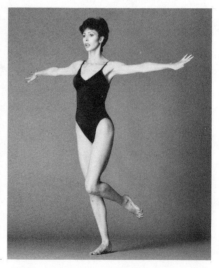

Jog. Arms out at shoulder height. Arms push front with palms front 4 counts.

Then, arms push back with palms back 4 counts.

13

JOG/HANDS TO SHOULDERS
(30 SECONDS)

Jog. Arms out at shoulder height. Keep your upper arms still as you bring hands to shoulders and back out straight.

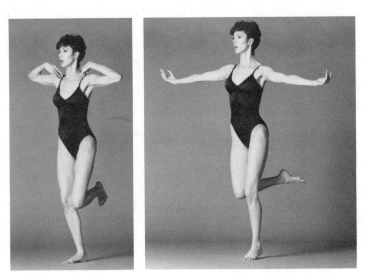

14

JOG/ REACH UP
(30 SECONDS)

Continue jogging. Both hands reach up above your head and down to your shoulders.

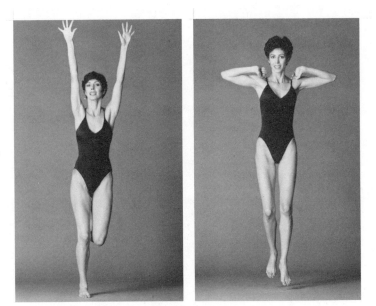

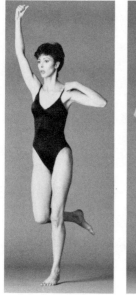
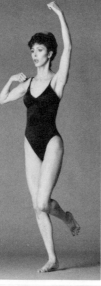

15 JOGGING PUNCHES (30 SECONDS)

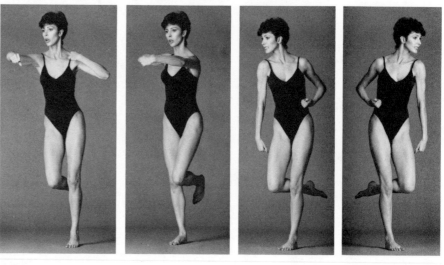

Jog in place. Hands punch up from the shoulders RIGHT and LEFT.

Then, hands punch front RIGHT and LEFT.

Then, continue to jog and punch hands down toward the floor RIGHT and LEFT.

16
JOG/ARMS CROSS IN AND OUT

(30 SECONDS)
Jog in place. Cross your hands in front of your body and out at shoulder height. Single counts.

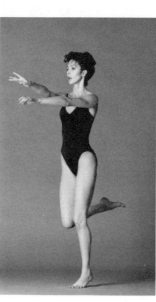
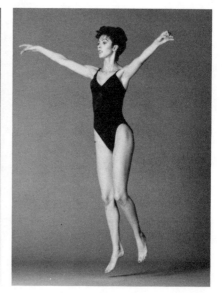

17
JOG/ DIAGONAL ARMS
(30 SECONDS)

Feet jog in place. Cross your hands low in front of your body, then up and out diagonally, alternating RIGHT and LEFT.

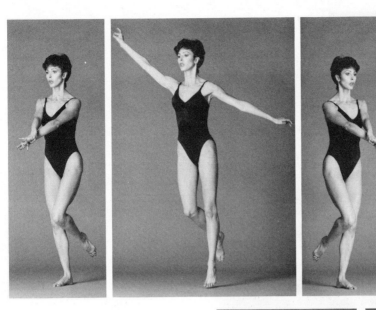

18
JOG/ STRAIGHT ARM SWINGS
(30 SECONDS)

Continue jogging. As RIGHT heel is down, RIGHT arm swings up. Then, as LEFT heel is down, LEFT arm swings up.

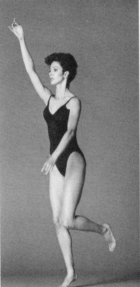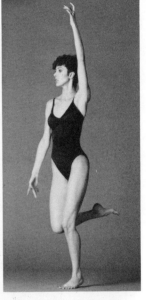

19
STEP KICK
(30 SECONDS)

RIGHT foot kicks out front as LEFT arm swings out front and RIGHT arm swings back. Then, LEFT foot kicks out as RIGHT arm swings front and LEFT arm swings back.

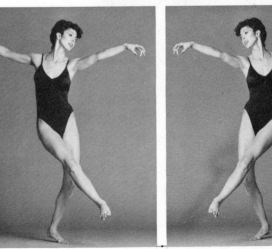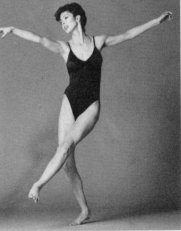

20
ELBOW-TO-KNEE LIFTS
(30 SECONDS)

Jog. Bring RIGHT knee up to meet LEFT elbow. Reverse, LEFT knee comes up to meet RIGHT elbow.

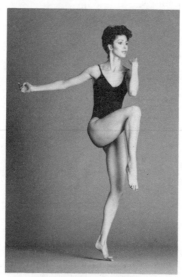

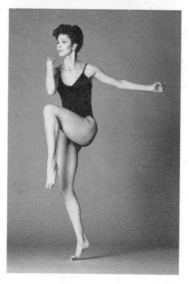

21
JUMP TOUCH
(30 SECONDS)

Feet jump together. Then alternate touching LEFT hand to RIGHT foot and RIGHT hand to LEFT foot in back of you, with free arm swinging over head.

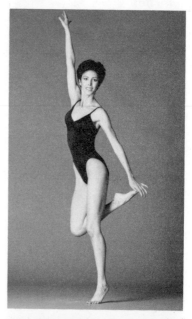

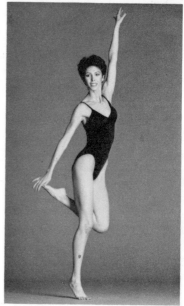

22
CROSS
JUMPS
(30 SECONDS)

Hands on waist. Jump. Feet cross at ankles and then out shoulder width. Alternate, crossing RIGHT then LEFT foot in front.

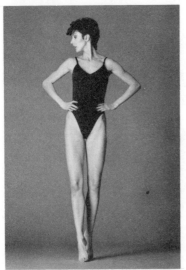

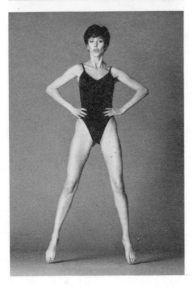

23
HALF-
JACKS
(30 SECONDS)

Jump up and out with your feet as arms swing up to shoulder height. Then, bring your feet together as arms come down to your sides.

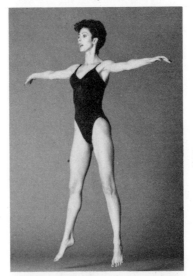

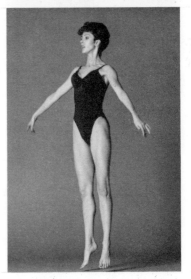

24

JUMPING
JACKS
(30 SECONDS)

Jump up and out with your feet as your arms swing up freely from the shoulders above your head. Then, bring your feet together as arms come down.

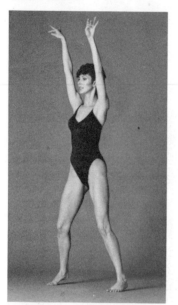

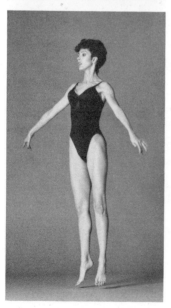

25

HEEL
JACKS
(30 SECONDS)

As you hop on LEFT foot, extend RIGHT foot out to side and touch RIGHT heel to floor, toes pointed upward. Thrust hip outward and swing arms above head. Alternate.

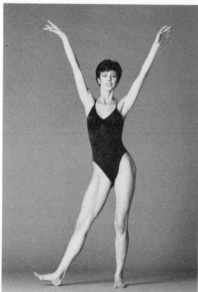

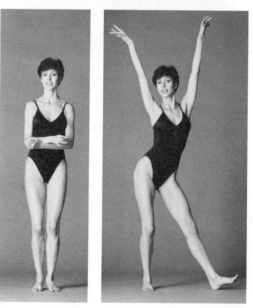

26
AEROBIC SIDE LUNGE
(30 SECONDS)

Lunge to the RIGHT. Both arms swing up straight to the RIGHT. Come center. Then lunge LEFT and swing both arms up to the LEFT.

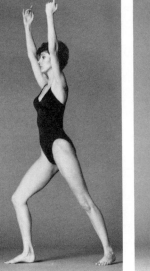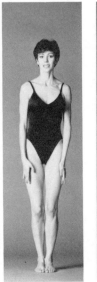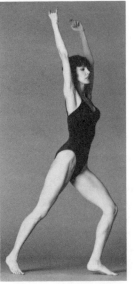

27
ONE-ARM LUNGE
(30 SECONDS)

Lunge body and RIGHT arm to the RIGHT as LEFT arm is bent in to body. Come center. Then, lunge LEFT as LEFT arm swings up straight.

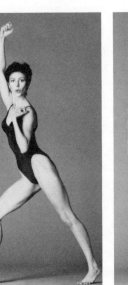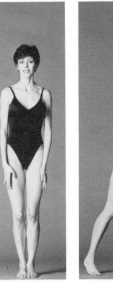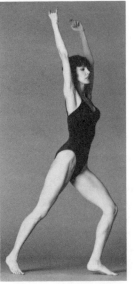

28
TWISTS
(60 SECONDS)

Jump with feet together and knees bent, twisting to the LEFT as arms cross the body at shoulder height to the RIGHT. Reverse to the RIGHT. Two counts on each side. Then, single twists.

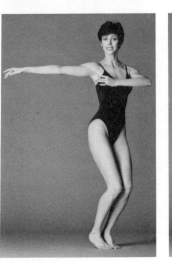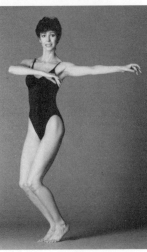

COOL-DOWN · 2 MINUTES
(Music—120 Beats Per Minute)

5
TWO-ARM STANDING LUNGE
(30 SECONDS)

Stand with feet shoulder width apart; arms at your sides. Slowly lunge body RIGHT 2 counts and LEFT two counts, cooling it down.

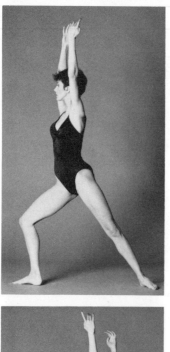

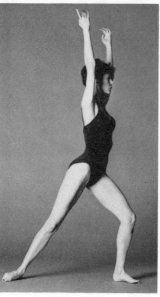

36
SHOULDER LEADS
(30 SECONDS)

Feet wide apart; legs bent; hands on knees. Twist your torso and press LEFT shoulder front 2 counts, then RIGHT shoulder front 2 counts.

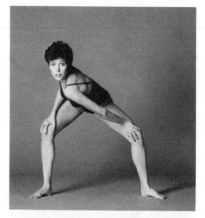

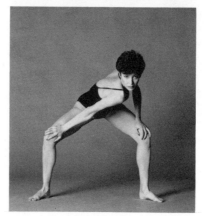

37
HEEL
RAISES &
PRESSES
(30 SECONDS)

Feet wide apart behind; hands apart on the floor in front of you; legs straight; back flat. Raise up and down on your toes in single counts, stretching your calves. Then, press your heels down and your chest toward the floor and hold 4 counts.

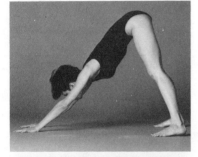

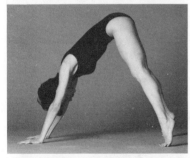

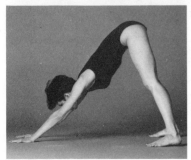

38
TENDON
STRETCH
(30 SECONDS)

Start with hands on the floor and feet and legs together and behind. Raise RIGHT heel up, bending RIGHT knee as you press LEFT heel to the floor for 2 counts. Reverse for the LEFT heel. Then, single counts. Then, heels to the floor and hold the stretch.

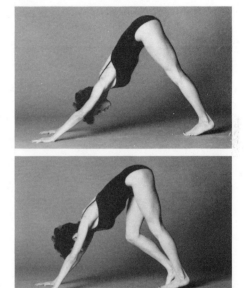

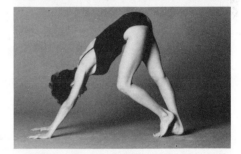

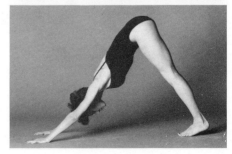

THE AEROBICISE WORKOUTS   115

WARM-UP · 3 MINUTES
(Music—126 Beats Per Minute)

3
SIDE STRETCHES
(30 SECONDS)

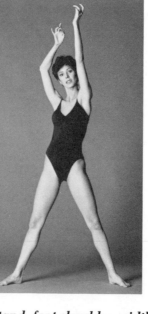
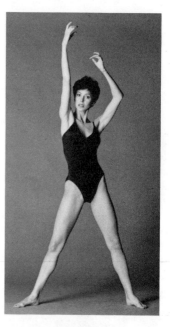

Stand; feet shoulder width apart. Reach up with your LEFT arm 2 counts, feeling the stretch in your LEFT side.

Reach up with your RIGHT arm 2 counts. Stretch up and out from the rib cage. Then, single counts LEFT and RIGHT.

4
BOW & ARROW
(30 SECONDS)

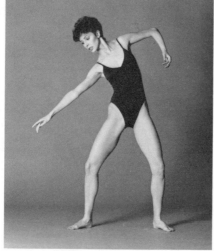
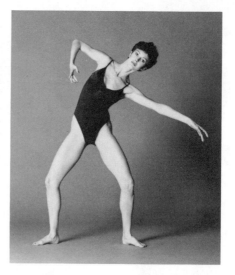

Stand with feet shoulder width apart; knees slightly bent. Starting to the RIGHT, reach RIGHT arm out straight as LEFT arm bows up. Feel the stretch in your LEFT side. Come back to center.

Reverse to the LEFT. Be sure to pull directly to the side, keeping your body front. Single counts RIGHT and LEFT.

5
TWO-ARM STANDING LUNGE
(30 SECONDS)

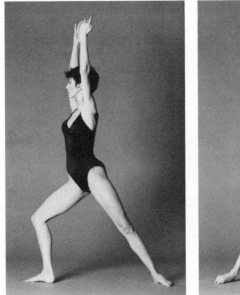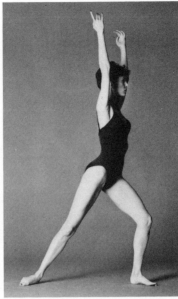

Feet wide apart; arms at sides; lunge body and RIGHT leg to the RIGHT as both arms swing up above head to the RIGHT. Come center.

Then, lunge LEFT. Keep it fluid. Use your arms for momentum.

6
ELBOW-TO-KNEE LUNGE
(30 SECONDS)

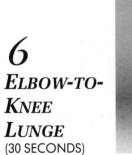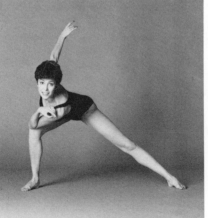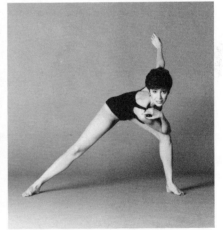

With a flat back, lunge to the RIGHT, reaching LEFT elbow to RIGHT knee and let your RIGHT arm swing up toward the ceiling.

Reverse to the LEFT, reaching RIGHT elbow to LEFT knee in single counts.

7
TOE
TOUCHES
(60 SECONDS)

Continue lunging, but reach LEFT elbow to the floor. Reverse with the RIGHT elbow. Reach down as far as you can. Keep your back flat.

With straight legs, alternate reaching LEFT hand to RIGHT foot and RIGHT hand to LEFT foot. Let your other arm swing up behind you. Single counts.

Now, reach LEFT hand behind RIGHT foot and RIGHT hand behind LEFT foot in single counts.

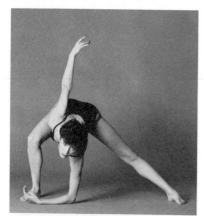 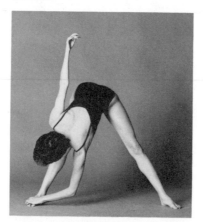 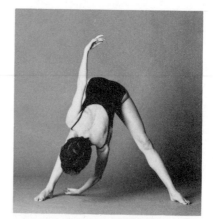

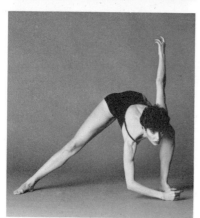 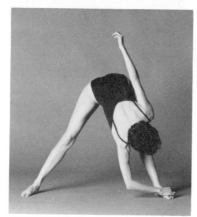 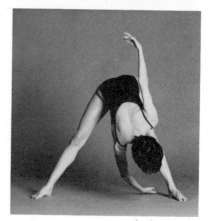

AEROBICS · 12 MINUTES
(Music—138 Beats Per Minute)

10
JOG
(30 SECONDS)

Pick up your feet lightly.
Land on the balls of your feet
and work it through the heels.
Keep it light.

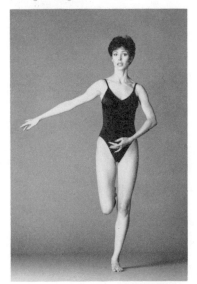

11
JOG/ARM CIRCLES
(30 SECONDS)

Feet jog in place. Arms out at
shoulder height. Circle arms
front with palms down 4
counts. Circle back with
palms up 4 counts.

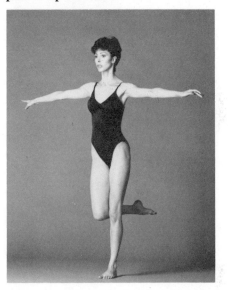

12
JOG/PUSH FRONT
(30 SECONDS)

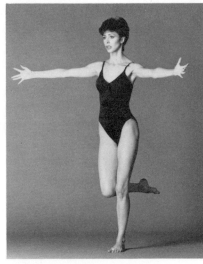 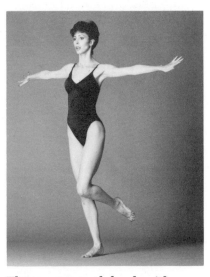

Jog. Arms out at shoulder
height. Arms push front with
palms front 4 counts.

Then, arms push back with
palms back 4 counts.

13
JOG/HANDS
TO
SHOULDERS
(30 SECONDS)

Jog. Arms out at shoulder height. Keep your upper arms still as you bring hands to shoulders and back out straight.

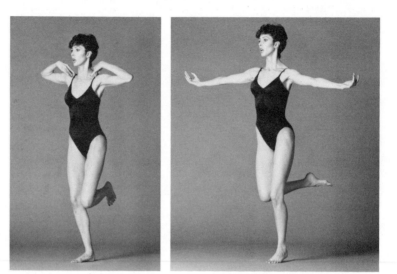

14
JOG/
REACH UP
(30 SECONDS)

Continue jogging. Both hands reach up above your head and down to your shoulders.

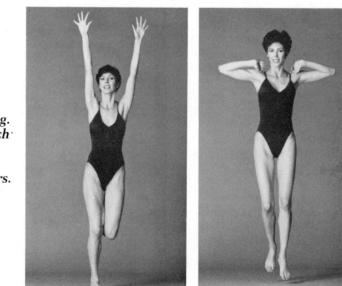

15 JOGGING PUNCHES (30 SECONDS)

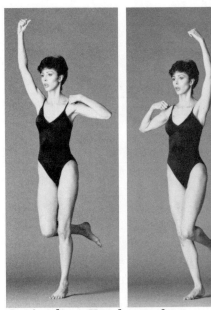 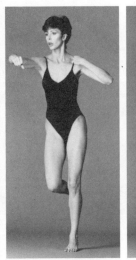 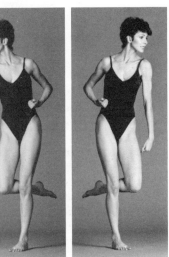

Jog in place. Hands punch up from the shoulders RIGHT *and* LEFT.

Then, hands punch front RIGHT *and* LEFT.

Then, continue to jog and punch hands down toward the floor RIGHT *and* LEFT.

16 JOG/ARMS CROSS IN AND OUT (30 SECONDS)

Jog in place. Cross your hands in front of your body and out at shoulder height. Single counts.

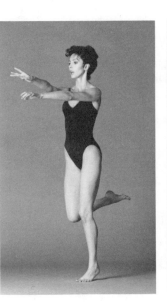 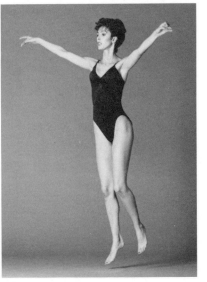

17
JOG/ DIAGONAL ARMS
(30 SECONDS)

Feet jog in place. Cross your hands low in front of your body, then up and out diagonally, alternating RIGHT *and* LEFT.

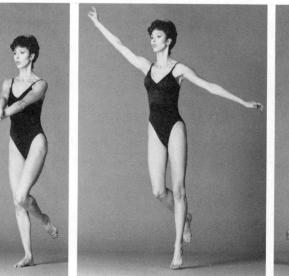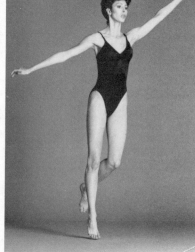

18
JOG/ STRAIGHT ARM SWINGS
(30 SECONDS)

Continue jogging. As RIGHT *heel is down,* RIGHT *arm swings up. Then, as* LEFT *heel is down,* LEFT *arm swings up.*

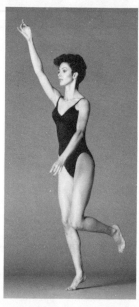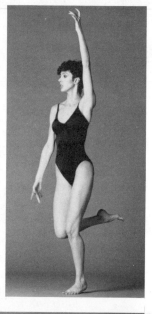

19
STEP KICK
(30 SECONDS)

RIGHT *foot kicks out front as* LEFT *arm swings out front and* RIGHT *arm swings back. Then,* LEFT *foot kicks out as* RIGHT *arm swings front and* LEFT *arm swings back.*

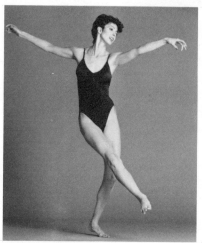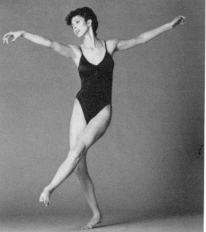

20
ELBOW TO KNEE LIFTS
(30 SECONDS)

Jog. Bring RIGHT knee up to meet LEFT elbow. Reverse, LEFT knee comes up to meet RIGHT elbow.

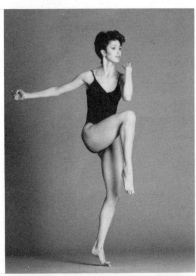

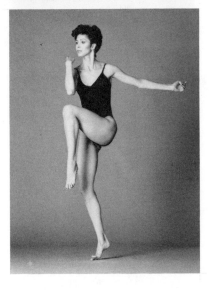

21
JUMP TOUCH
(30 SECONDS)

Feet jump together. Then alternate touching LEFT hand to RIGHT foot and RIGHT hand to LEFT foot in back of you, with free arm swinging over head.

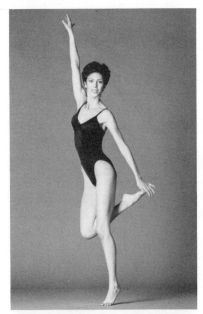

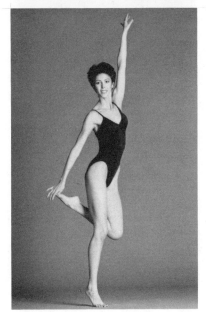

22
CROSS
JUMPS
(30 SECONDS)

Hands on waist. Jump. Feet cross at ankles and then out shoulder width. Alternate, crossing RIGHT then LEFT foot in front.

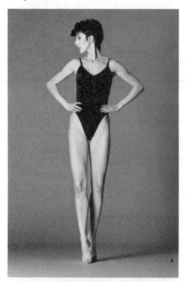

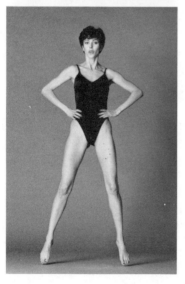

23
HALF-
JACKS
(30 SECONDS)

Jump up and out with your feet as arms swing up to shoulder height. Then, bring your feet together as arms come down to your sides.

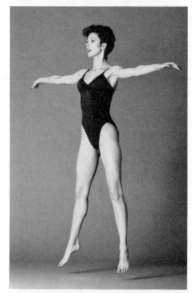

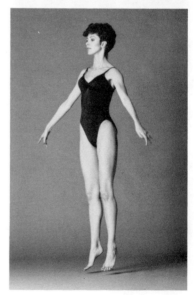

24

JUMPING JACKS
(30 SECONDS)

Jump up and out with your feet as your arms swing up freely from the shoulders above your head. Then, bring your feet together as arms come down.

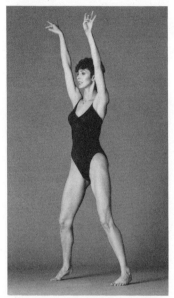

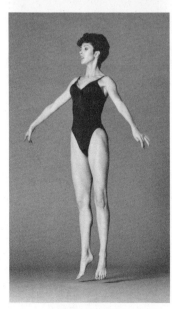

25

HEEL JACKS
(30 SECONDS)

As you hop on LEFT foot, extend RIGHT foot out to side and touch RIGHT heel to floor, toes pointed upward. Thrust hip outward and swing arms above head. Alternate.

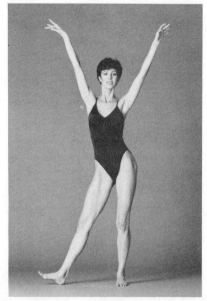

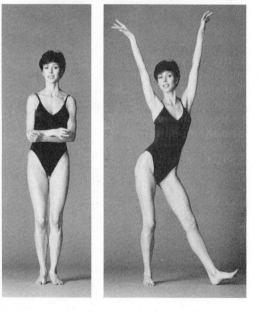

26
AEROBIC
SIDE
LUNGE
(30 SECONDS)

*Lunge to the
RIGHT. Both arms
swing up straight
to the RIGHT.
Come center.
Then lunge LEFT
and swing both
arms up to
the LEFT.*

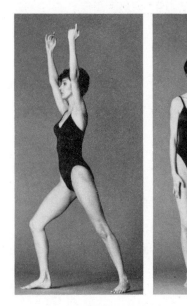
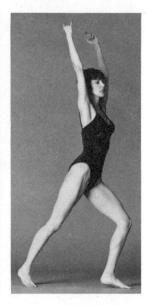

27
ONE-ARM
LUNGE
(30 SECONDS)

*Lunge body and
RIGHT arm to
the RIGHT as
LEFT arm is
bent in to body.
Come center.
Then, lunge
LEFT as LEFT
arm swings
up straight.*

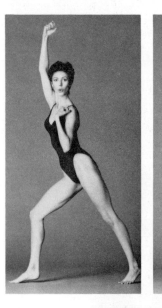
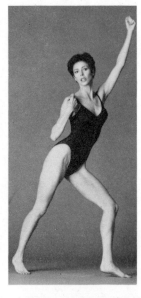

28
TWISTS
(60 SECONDS)

*Jump with feet together and
knees bent, twisting to the
LEFT as arms cross the body at
shoulder height to the RIGHT.
Reverse to the RIGHT. Two
counts on each side. Then,
single twists.*

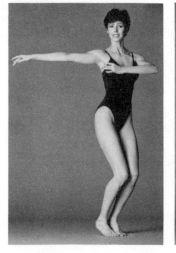
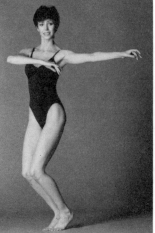

29

ARM
MEETS
THE LEG
(30 SECONDS)

Hop on one foot as you swing other leg out to side; feet move side to side. As RIGHT arm swings up straight from the shoulder, LEFT arm is down at your side to meet extended LEFT leg. As LEFT arm swings up, RIGHT arm meets RIGHT leg.

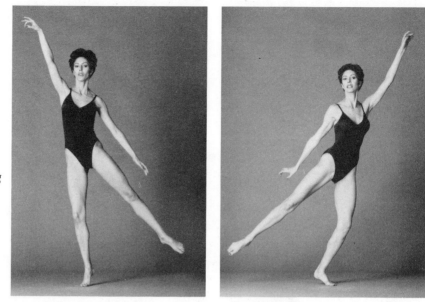

30

HAND
TO HEEL
(30 SECONDS)

Jog. LEFT heel comes up to meet LEFT hand. Then, reverse. RIGHT heel meets RIGHT hand.

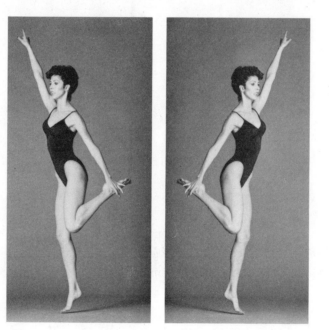

31
WILD
JUMPS
(30 SECONDS)

Jump with feet together. Then jump and bring heels up and close to buttocks.

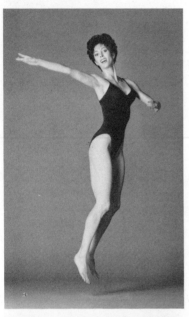

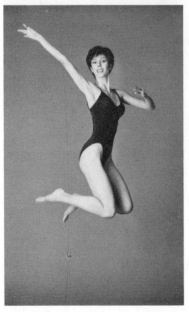

32
JOG/HANDS
CROSS LOW
(30 SECONDS)

Jog. Hands cross low in front of body and low behind.

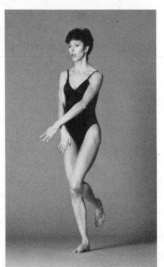

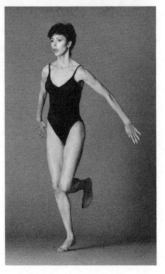

COOL-DOWN · 3 MINUTES
(Music—126 Beats Per Minute)

5
TWO-ARM STANDING LUNGE
(30 SECONDS)

Stand with feet shoulder width apart, arms at your sides. Slowly lunge body RIGHT 2 counts and LEFT 2 counts, cooling it down.

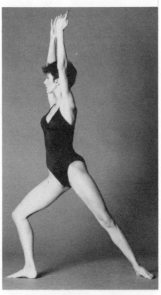

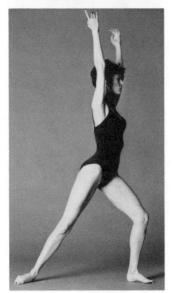

36
SHOULDER LEADS
(30 SECONDS)

Feet wide apart; legs bent; hands on knees. Twist your torso and press LEFT shoulder front 2 counts, then RIGHT shoulder front 2 counts.

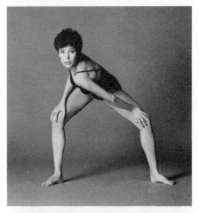

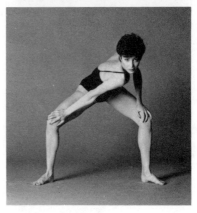

37

HEEL RAISES & PRESSES
(30 SECONDS)

Feet wide apart; hands apart on the floor in front of you; legs straight; back flat. Raise up and down on your toes in single counts, stretching your calves. Then, press your heels down and your chest toward the floor and hold 4 counts.

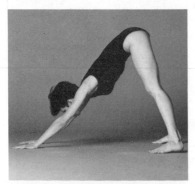

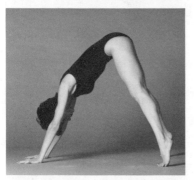

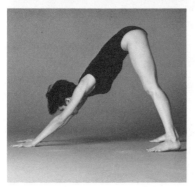

38

TENDON STRETCH
(30 SECONDS)

Start with hands on the floor and feet and legs together behind. Raise RIGHT heel up, bending RIGHT knee as you press LEFT heel to the floor for 2 counts. Reverse for the LEFT heel. Then, single counts. Then, heels to the floor and hold the stretch.

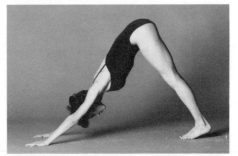

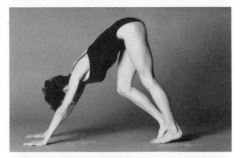

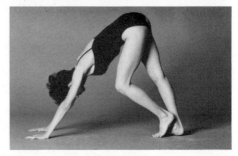

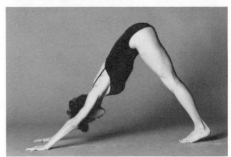

39
SHOULDER STAND TO PLOUGH
(60 SECONDS)

Lie on your back. Roll your feet up, legs straight, in the air. Support your back with your hands. Then, extend your legs straight out behind you. Arms may be out to the side or keep them behind your back for support. Then, slowly roll down to the floor.

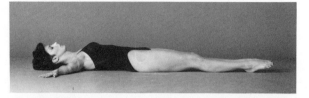

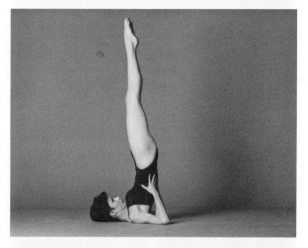

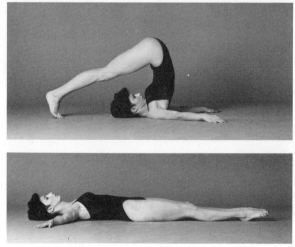

WARM-UP · 4 MINUTES
(Music—132 Beats Per Minute)

3

SIDE STRETCHES
(30 SECONDS)

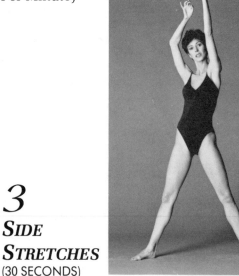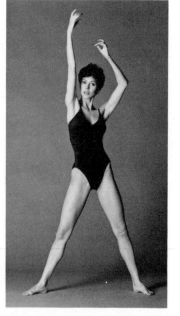

Stand; feet shoulder width apart. Reach up with your LEFT arm 2 counts, feeling the stretch in your LEFT side.

Reach up with your RIGHT arm 2 counts. Stretch up and out from the rib cage. Then, single counts LEFT and RIGHT.

4

BOW & ARROW
(30 SECONDS)

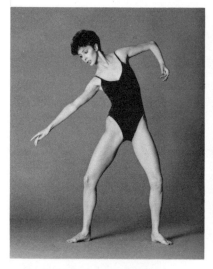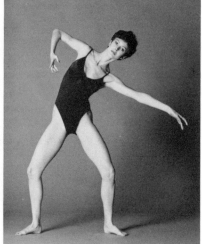

Stand with feet shoulder width apart; knees slightly bent. Starting to the RIGHT, reach RIGHT arm out straight as LEFT arm bows up. Feel the stretch in your LEFT side. Come back to center.

Reverse to the LEFT. Be sure to pull directly to the side, keeping your body front. Single counts RIGHT and LEFT.

5
TWO-ARM STANDING LUNGE
(30 SECONDS)

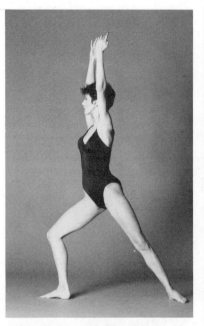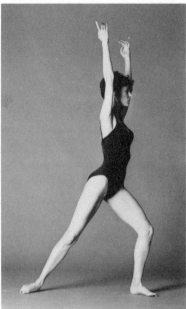

Feet wide apart; arms at sides; lunge body and RIGHT leg to the RIGHT as both arms swing up above head to the RIGHT. Come center.

Then, lunge LEFT. Keep it fluid. Use your arms for momentum.

6
ELBOW-TO-KNEE LUNGE
(30 SECONDS)

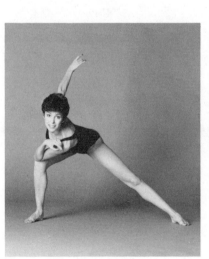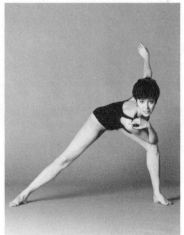

With a flat back, lunge to the RIGHT, reaching LEFT elbow to RIGHT knee and let your RIGHT arm swing up toward the ceiling.

Reverse to the LEFT, reaching RIGHT elbow to LEFT knee in single counts.

TOE TOUCHES
(60 SECONDS)

Continue lunging, but reach LEFT elbow to the floor. Reverse with the RIGHT elbow. Reach down as far as you can. Keep your back flat.

With straight legs, alternate reaching LEFT hand to RIGHT foot and RIGHT hand to LEFT foot. Let your other arm swing up behind you. Single counts.

Now, reach LEFT hand behind RIGHT foot and RIGHT hand behind LEFT foot in single counts.

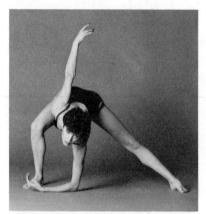
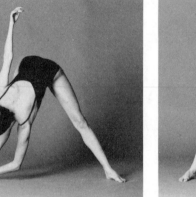
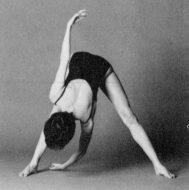

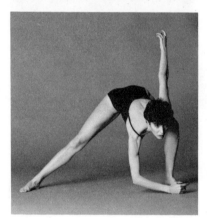
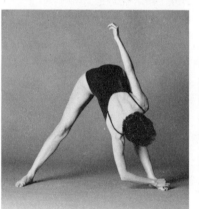
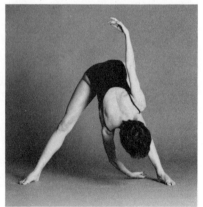

8
FLAT 2 PUSH-
THROUGH
(30 SECONDS)

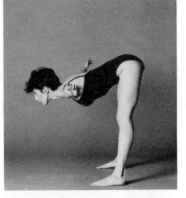 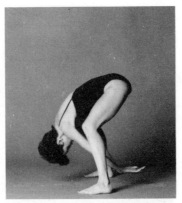

Feet wide apart; back flat, arms out parallel to the ground. Gently bounce your back toward the floor 2 counts.

Then, bend knees and push hands through legs 2 counts.

9
STANDING
STRETCH
(30 SECONDS)

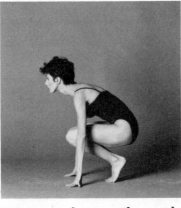 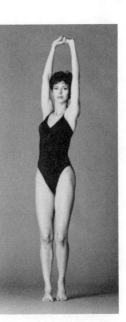

Bring your feet together and hands on the floor.

Gently roll up; stand tall and stretch it out.

AEROBICS · 14 MINUTES
(Music—144 Beats Per Minute)

10
JOG
(30 SECONDS)

*Pick up your feet lightly.
Land on the balls of your feet
and work it through the heels.
Keep it light.*

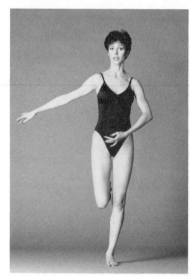

11
JOG/ARM CIRCLES
(30 SECONDS)

*Feet jog in place. Arms out at
shoulder height. Circle arms
front with palms down 4
counts. Circle back with
palms up 4 counts.*

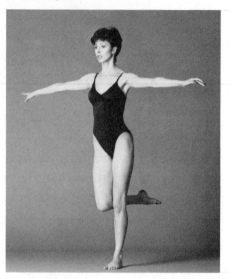

12
JOG/PUSH FRONT
(30 SECONDS)

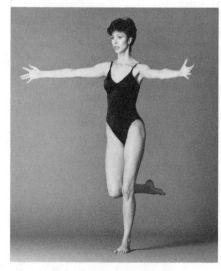
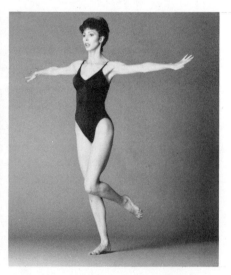

*Jog. Arms out at shoulder
height. Arms push front with
palms front 4 counts.*

*Then, arms push back with
palms back 4 counts.*

13
JOG/HANDS TO SHOULDERS
(30 SECONDS)

Jog. Arms out at shoulder height. Keep your upper arms still as you bring hands to shoulders and back out straight.

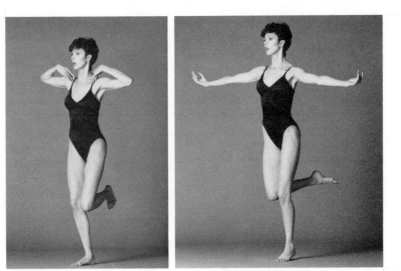

14
JOG/ REACH UP
(30 SECONDS)

Continue jogging. Both hands reach up above your head and down to your shoulders.

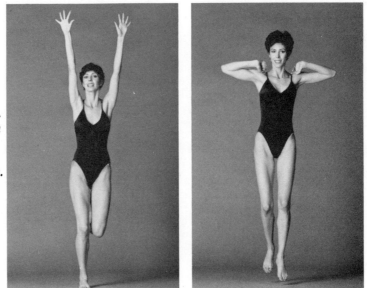

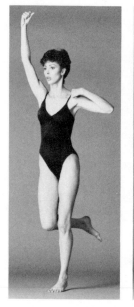
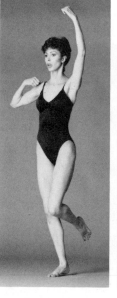

15 JOGGING PUNCHES (60 SECONDS)

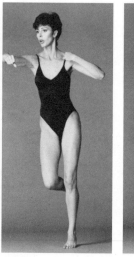
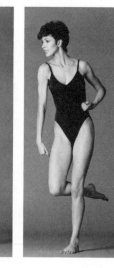
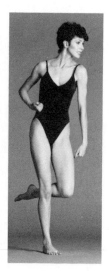

Jog in place. Hands punch up from the shoulders RIGHT and LEFT.

Then, hands punch front RIGHT and LEFT.

Then, continue to jog and punch hands down toward the floor RIGHT and LEFT.

16
JOG/ARMS CROSS IN AND OUT
(30 SECONDS)

Jog in place. Cross your hands in front of your body and out at shoulder height. Single counts.

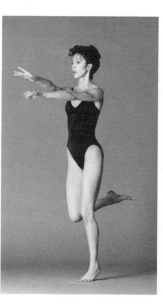
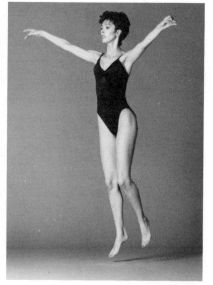

17

JOG/ DIAGONAL ARMS

(30 SECONDS)

Feet jog in place. Cross your hands low in front of your body, then up and out diagonally, alternating RIGHT and LEFT.

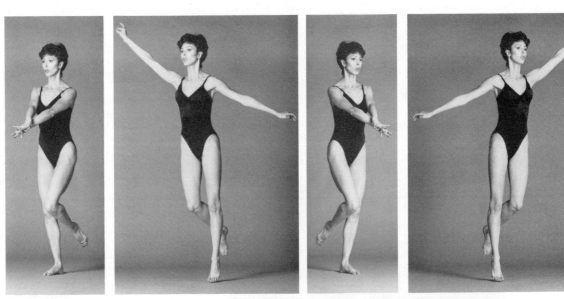

18

JOG/ STRAIGHT ARM SWINGS

(30 SECONDS)

Continue jogging. As RIGHT heel is down, RIGHT arm swings up. Then, as LEFT heel is down, LEFT arm swings up.

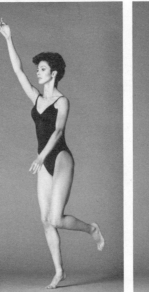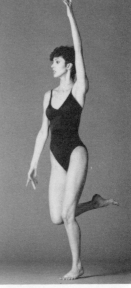

19

STEP KICK

(30 SECONDS)

RIGHT foot kicks out front as LEFT arm swings out front and RIGHT arm swings back. Then, LEFT foot kicks out as RIGHT arm swings front and LEFT arm swings back.

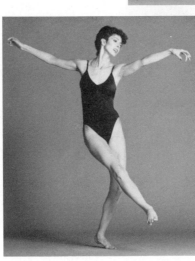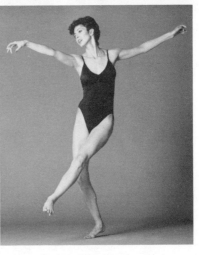

20

ELBOW-TO-KNEE LIFTS
(30 SECONDS)

Jog. Bring RIGHT knee up to meet LEFT elbow. Reverse, LEFT knee comes up to meet RIGHT elbow.

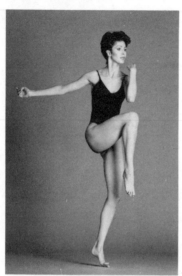

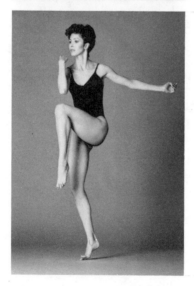

21

JUMP TOUCH
(30 SECONDS)

Feet jump together. Then alternate touching LEFT hand to RIGHT foot and RIGHT hand to LEFT foot in back of you, with free arm swinging over head.

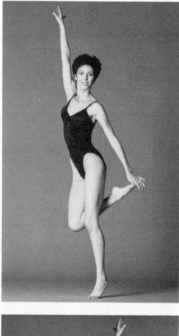

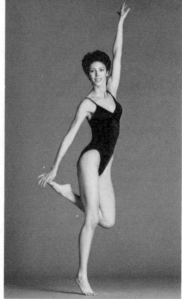

22
CROSS
JUMPS
(30 SECONDS)

Hands on waist. Jump. Feet cross at ankles and then out shoulder width. Alternate, crossing RIGHT then LEFT foot in front.

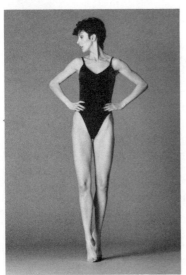

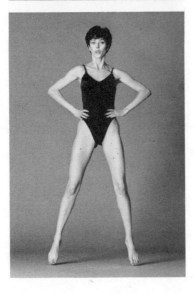

23
HALF-
JACKS
(30 SECONDS)

Jump up and out with your feet as arms swing up to shoulder height. Then, bring your feet together as arms come down to your sides.

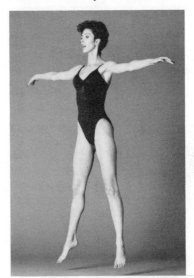

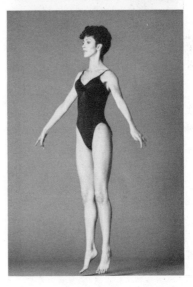

24

JUMPING
JACKS
(30 SECONDS)

*Jump up and out with your
feet as your arms swing up
freely from the shoulders
above your head. Then, bring
your feet together as arms
come down.*

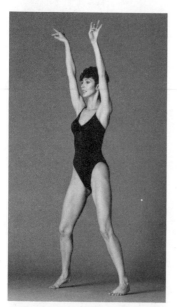

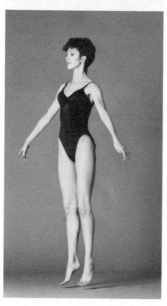

25

HEEL
JACKS
(30 SECONDS)

As you hop on LEFT *foot,
extend* RIGHT *foot out to side
and touch* RIGHT *heel to floor,
toes pointed upward. Thrust
hip outward and swing arms
above head. Alternate.*

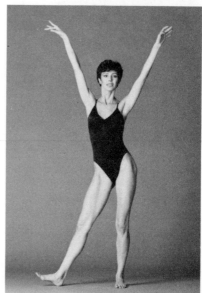

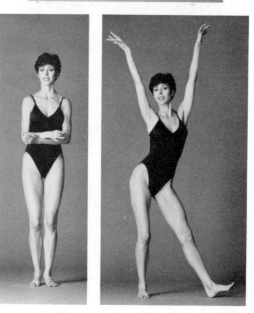

26
Aerobic Side Lunge
(30 SECONDS)

Lunge to the RIGHT. Both arms swing up straight to the RIGHT. Come center. Then lunge LEFT and swing both arms up to the left.

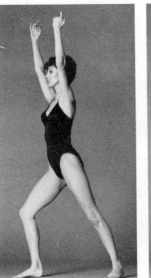 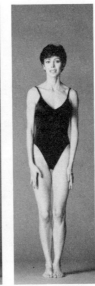 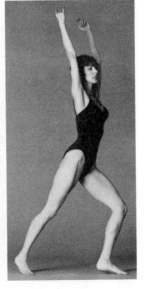

27
One Arm Lunge
(30 SECONDS)

Lunge body and RIGHT arm to the RIGHT as LEFT arm is bent in to body. Come center. Then, lunge LEFT as LEFT arm swings up straight.

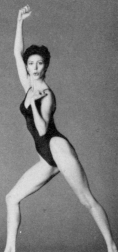 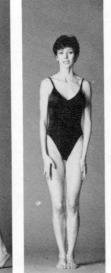 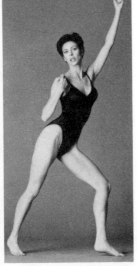

28
Twists
(60 SECONDS)

Jump with feet together and knees bent, twisting to the LEFT as arms cross the body at shoulder height to the RIGHT. Reverse to the RIGHT. Two counts on each side. Then, single twists.

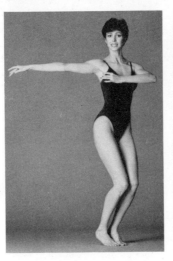 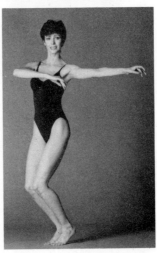

29
ARM
MEETS
THE LEG
(30 SECONDS)

Hop on one foot as you swing other leg out to side; feet move side to side. As RIGHT arm swings up straight from the shoulder, LEFT arm is down at your side to meet extended LEFT leg. As LEFT arm swings up, RIGHT arm meets RIGHT leg.

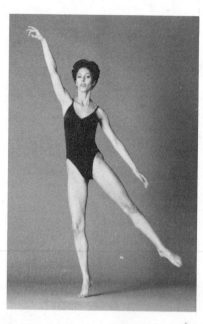 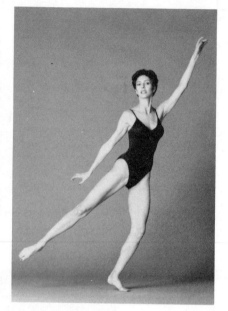

30
HAND TO
HEEL
(30 SECONDS)

Jog. LEFT heel comes up to meet LEFT hand. Then, reverse, RIGHT heel meets RIGHT hand.

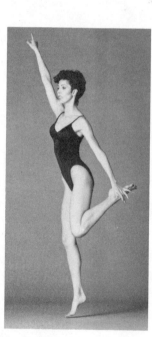 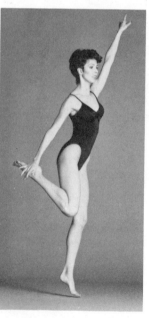

31
WILD JUMPS
(30 SECONDS)

Jump with feet together. Then jump and bring heels up and close to buttocks.

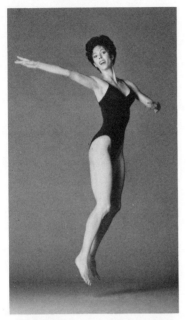

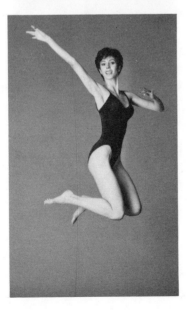

32
JOG/HANDS
CROSS LOW
(30 SECONDS)

Jog. Hands cross low in front of body and low behind.

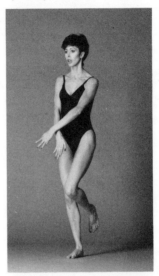

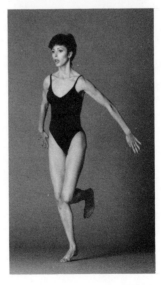

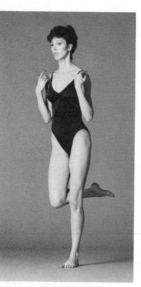

33

JOG/ARM RELEASE
(30 SECONDS)

Slowly jog in place as lower arms bend in to chest and down to your sides.

10

JOG
(60 SECONDS)

Slowly jog in place, cooling it down.

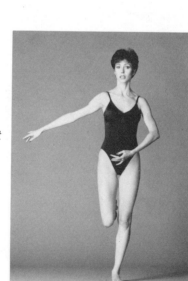

COOL-DOWN · 3 MINUTES
(Music—132 Beats Per Minute)

5
TWO-ARM STANDING LUNGE
(30 SECONDS)

Stand with feet shoulder width apart; arms at your sides. Slowly lunge body RIGHT 2 counts and LEFT 2 counts.

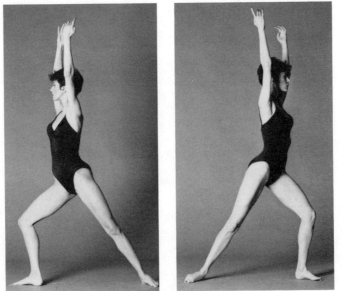

37
HEEL RAISES & PRESSES
(30 SECONDS)

Feet wide apart; hands apart on the floor in front of you; legs straight; back flat. Raise up and down on your toes in single counts, stretching your calves. Then, press your heels down and your chest toward the floor and hold 4 counts.

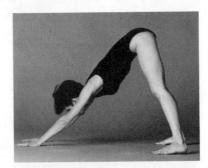

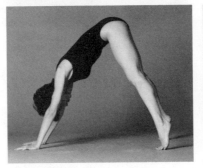

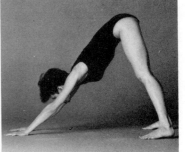

38
TENDON STRETCH
(30 SECONDS)

Start with hands on the floor and feet and legs together behind. Raise RIGHT heel up, bending RIGHT knee as you press LEFT heel to the floor for 2 counts. Reverse for the LEFT heel. Then, single counts. Then, heels to the floor and hold the stretch.

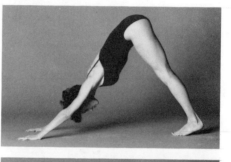

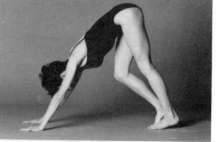

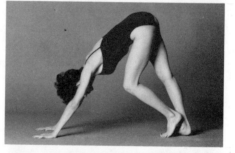

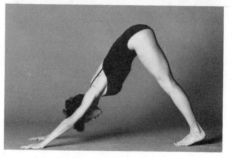

39

SHOULDER STAND TO PLOUGH
(60 SECONDS)

Lie on your back. Roll your feet up, legs straight, in the air. Support your back with your hands. Then, extend your legs straight out behind you. Arms may be out to the side or keep them behind your back for support. Then, slowly roll down to the floor.

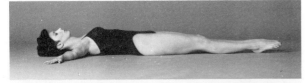

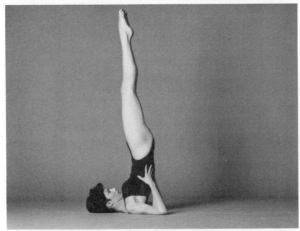

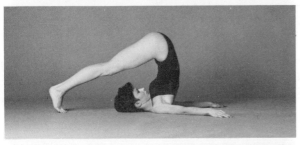

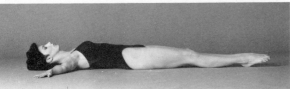

40

REACH OVER
(30 SECONDS)

Sit up; arms out at shoulder height; stomach held in. With a flat back, reach over toward ankles as far as you can, bringing your head to your knees. Hold for a count of 10.

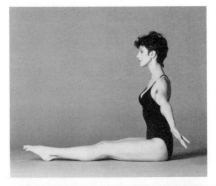

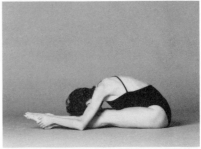

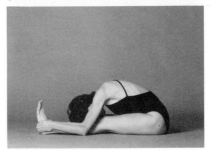

Point and flex your feet.

CHAPTER SIX

THE EXTRA WORKOUTS: TONE-UPS

This chapter covers all the special areas not included in the primary workouts. You can add them to the other workouts, before the aerobics portion, to give yourself a longer routine or just to add variety. There is no such thing as "spot-reducing." You can, however, "spot-tone," shape and firm specific muscles. Remember, it is only through aerobics that you are going to burn fat. These extra workouts are good tone-ups but do not take the place of aerobics for cardiovascular fitness.

ARMS WORKOUT

This workout was designed to strengthen, tone, and shape the muscles of your arms, chest, and back. Specifically, it works the *biceps* and *triceps*, the muscles on your upper arms, which work together to bend your elbows and control your forearms; your *deltoids*, or shoulder muscles, which control the raising and lowering of your arms; your *pectoralis major*, which extends from your collarbone down the outside of your breastbone and across your seventh rib; the *pectoralis minor*, which lies under the pectoralis major and helps move the shoulder and upper arm; the *trapezius*, which extends from the base of the skull to the vertebrae at the middle of your back; the *tenes major* and *minor* on your upper arm, which help extend and move the arms; and the *latissimus dorsi*, located on your back, which pull the arms down, turn them inward, and help you pull them behind your back.

Use the music listed for tone-ups in Chapter 7.

41

ELBOW EXTENSIONS
(30 SECONDS)
(TRICEPS)

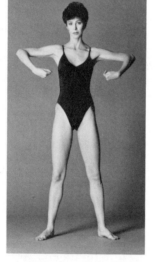 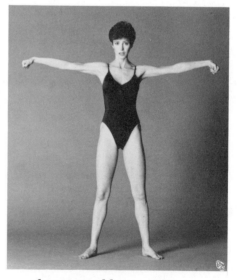

Stand with feet shoulder width apart; stomach held in; hips tucked under. Bring lower arms in toward your body with clenched fists . . .

. . . then extend lower arms out to shoulder height in a pendulum movement. Move only your lower arms, keeping shoulders and upper arms still. In and out make up one count.

42
DIAGONAL ARM STRETCHES
(30 SECONDS)
(PECTORALS)

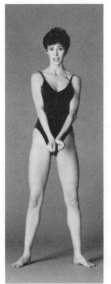

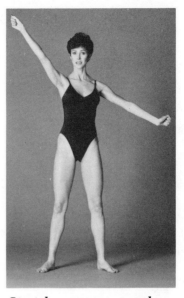

Stand with feet shoulder width apart; stomach held in; hips tucked under. Fists are clenched low in front of your body.

Stretch RIGHT arm up above your head and back as LEFT arm swings low to the back.

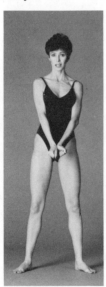

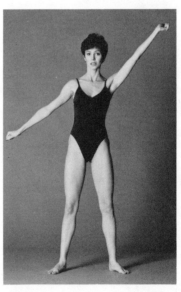

Arms come back to center.

Stretch LEFT arm up above your head and back as RIGHT arm swings low to the back. Feel the stretch across your chest.

43
SCISSORS
(30 SECONDS)

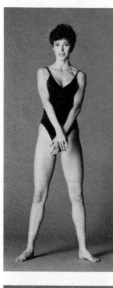

Stand with feet shoulder width apart; hips tucked under. Cross RIGHT arm over LEFT in a scissoring motion up above your head in 4 counts . . .

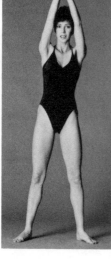

. . . and down to starting position in 4 counts. Keep your arms straight and tight and your stomach muscles in.

44
TRICEP EXTENSIONS
(30 SECONDS)
(TRICEPS)

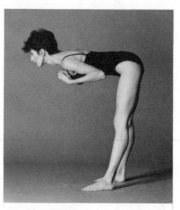

Stand with feet a little more than hip distance apart. Bend over at the waist into a flat back; fists are clenched and arms are close to your sides.

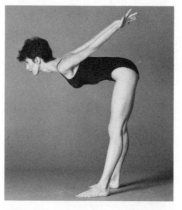

Extend your arms and hands straight up behind your back, stretching your fingers open, then back in toward your body. In and out make up one count.

45
PUSH-UPS
(30 SECONDS)

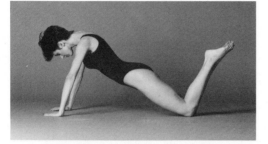

Get down on the floor. Hands are spread out in front of you shoulder width apart, supporting your upper body. Knees are on the floor, legs bent in a V and slightly apart. Keep head, back and buttocks on the same angle. Inhale in the up position . . .

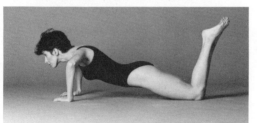

. . . and exhale as you bend your elbows and bring your chest toward the floor. Keep your stomach muscles tight. NOTE: Doing this with your hands out at shoulder width works your pectoral muscles. Done with hands closer together, this is good for your tricep muscles. Try it both ways.

WAIST WORKOUT

This workout was designed to strengthen, tone, and shape the muscles of your waist and back areas: specifically, your *intercostals*, or rib muscles, which raise and lower the rib cage, making it possible for you to breathe; your *external* and *internal oblique* muscles, located at your waist, which make it possible for you to bend forward and backward; and your *latissimus dorsi*, those muscles near the side of your back.

Use the music listed for tone-ups in Chapter 7.

46
WAIST REACHES
(30 SECONDS)
(OBLIQUES AND WAIST)

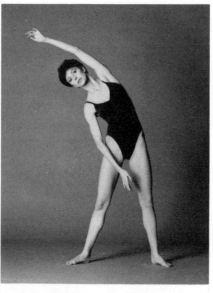 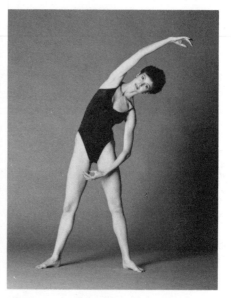

Stand with feet more than shoulder width apart and slightly turned out. Starting to the RIGHT, reach LEFT arm over your ear as RIGHT arm curves low in front of your body. Pull directly to the side for 2 counts, keeping your body and hips front.

Then, reverse with the RIGHT arm reaching over your head to the LEFT. Keep your stomach muscles in and remember to breathe out. Then, single counts RIGHT and LEFT.

47
BEHIND REACHES
(30 SECONDS)

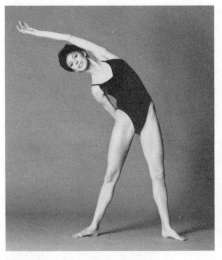

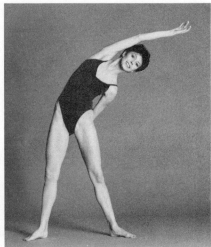

Stand with feet more than shoulder width apart and slightly turned out. Reach LEFT arm over head and RIGHT arm behind your hips.

Reverse, reaching RIGHT arm over head and LEFT arm behind your hips. Keep your stomach and buttocks muscles tight and your weight evenly distributed over both feet.

48
ADVANCED SIDE STRETCHES
(30 SECONDS)

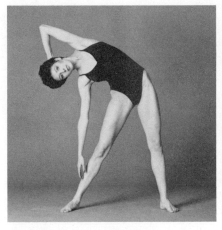

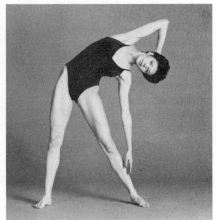

Stand with feet shoulder width apart and slightly turned out. Place LEFT hand behind your head and reach RIGHT hand down RIGHT calf as far as you can. Pull directly to the side, getting a good stretch.

Then, reverse with RIGHT hand behind your head and LEFT hand reaching down LEFT calf.

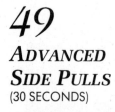

49
ADVANCED
SIDE PULLS
(30 SECONDS)

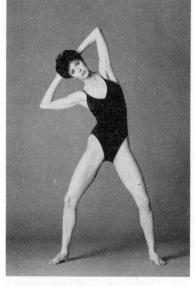 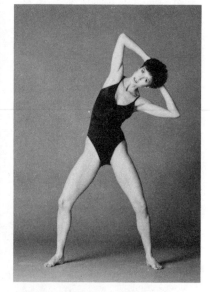

Stand with feet shoulder width apart; knees slightly bent; stomach held in; hips tucked under; hands are crossed behind your head. Pull to your RIGHT, feeling the stretch in your LEFT side.

Then, pull to your LEFT, feeling the stretch in your RIGHT side. Be sure to keep your body front, pulling directly to the side.

50
WAIST
TWISTS
(30 SECONDS)

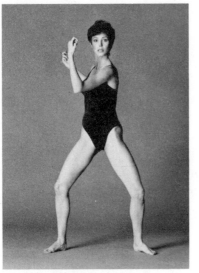
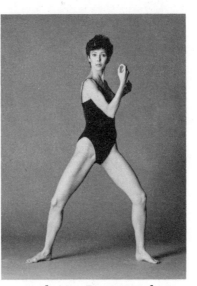

Stand with feet planted firmly on the floor, knees bent. Arms are bent up; hips are still. Twist from the waist up only, RIGHT . . .

. . . and LEFT. Be sure to keep your lower body front, working the waist only.

51
WAIST
PUNCHES
(30 SECONDS)

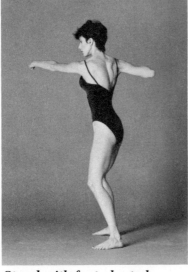
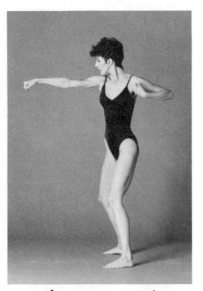

Stand with feet planted firmly on the floor, knees bent. Hips are still. Throw hands out in front of you in a punching motion LEFT . . .

. . . and RIGHT as you twist from the waist up only. Keep your weight even over both feet.

STOMACH WORKOUT

This workout was designed to firm, tone, and strengthen your abdominal muscles. Specifically, this works on the *oblique* muscles located where your "love handles" can be found.

Be sure to keep your lower back pressed to the floor for the exercises that are done on your back. Also, be sure you are using your abdominal muscles. That means, keep them held in. You'll find that the more you think about keeping your abdominal muscles pulled in, whatever you are doing, the better you'll look and the stronger they'll become.

Use the music listed for tone-ups in Chapter 7.

52
SIT-UPS
(60 SECONDS)

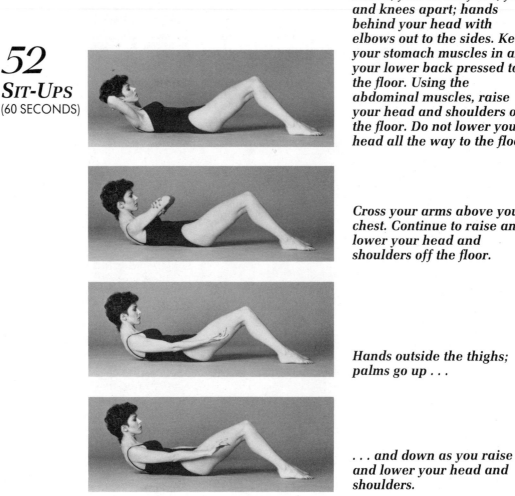

Lie on your back; knees raised; feet on the floor; feet and knees apart; hands behind your head with elbows out to the sides. Keep your stomach muscles in and your lower back pressed to the floor. Using the abdominal muscles, raise your head and shoulders off the floor. Do not lower your head all the way to the floor.

Cross your arms above your chest. Continue to raise and lower your head and shoulders off the floor.

Hands outside the thighs; palms go up . . .

. . . and down as you raise and lower your head and shoulders.

53
ABDOMINAL RELEASE
(30 SECONDS)

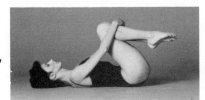

Lie flat on your back. Relax your head to the floor. Hug your knees in to your chest, and hold for a count of 10. Release all the tension in your abdominal muscles.

54
TRICYCLE
(30 SECONDS)

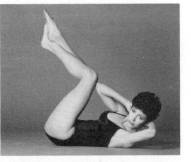 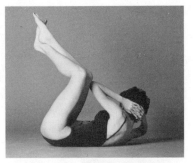

Lie on your back with your knees pulled up toward your chest and feet crossed at the ankles. With your hands clasped behind your head and head raised slightly off the floor, bring RIGHT elbow to LEFT knee, lifting your shoulders and chest off the floor . . .

. . . and LEFT elbow to RIGHT knee. Keep your stomach muscles in and your lower back pressed to the floor.

55
BICYCLE
(30 SECONDS)

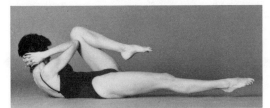

Lie on your back, hands clasped behind your head. Extend your RIGHT leg low off the floor with toes pointed. Twist your body, touching RIGHT elbow to LEFT knee as it comes up to your chest.

Then, touch LEFT elbow to RIGHT knee as it bends in to your chest. LEFT leg is low off the floor. Keep your head and shoulders off the floor, your stomach muscles in and your lower back pressed to the ground. Repeat, alternating legs in a continuous motion.

56 UNICYCLE
(30 SECONDS)

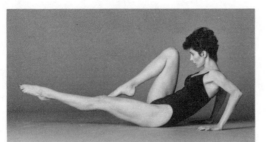

Sit on your buttocks, hands on floor behind, elbows bent, legs out straight off the floor. Alternate touching RIGHT foot to LEFT knee, which is low off the floor, in 2 counts . . .

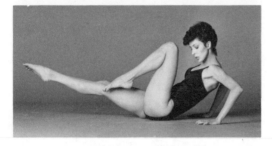

. . . and LEFT foot to RIGHT knee in 2 counts. Stomach muscles in. Then single counts RIGHT and LEFT.

57 STRAIGHT LEG BICYCLE
(30 SECONDS)

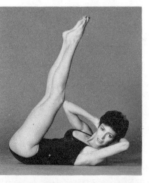

Lie on your back, hands clasped behind your head. Extend your legs straight in the air together. Twist your shoulders off the floor as you touch RIGHT elbow to LEFT knee . . .

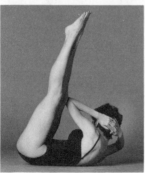

. . . and LEFT elbow to RIGHT knee. Keep your stomach muscles in and your head and shoulders off the floor.

58
KNEES
TO CHEST
(30 SECONDS)

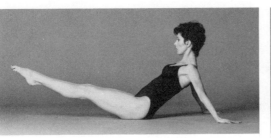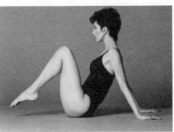

Sit on your buttocks, arms straight with hands stretched out behind, legs out straight and together off the floor.

Bring both knees in to your chest and out straight. Keep your stomach muscles tight and don't let your legs touch the floor.

59
WIDE
SCISSORS
(30 SECONDS)

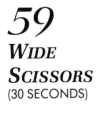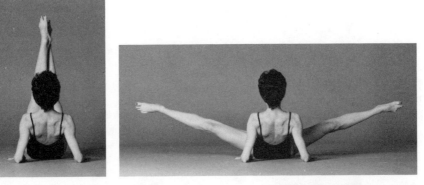

Sit on your buttocks, resting back on your elbows. Cross feet up in the air at the ankles . . .

. . . and extend them out in a wide V. Repeat the motion in and out. Don't let your feet touch the floor.

53
ABDOMINAL
RELEASE

Relax your head to the floor. Hug your knees in to your chest, and hold for a count of 10. Release all the tension in your abdominal muscles.

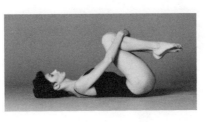

BUTTOCKS WORKOUT

This workout was designed to strengthen, firm, and tone the muscles of your buttocks: specifically, your *gluteus maximus*, located on the back of your buttocks; the *gluteus medius* and *minimus*, located on the front of your upper pelvic area (these three muscles help move the hip joints in all of your running and climbing activities), and the *biceps femoris*, located on your outer thigh.

Strong, firm buttocks muscles fight our natural enemy—gravity—and leave you looking lean and mean.

Use the music listed for tone-ups in Chapter 7.

60
HIP ROLLS
(30 SECONDS)
(PROMOTES TRUNK FLEXIBILITY; TONES AND TIGHTENS ABDOMEN)

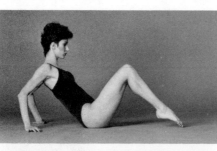

Sit on your buttocks and lean back slightly; knees together and bent; heels off the floor; hands behind and apart, supporting your weight on your hips.

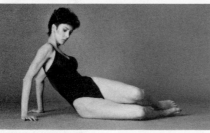

Rotate your knees to the RIGHT, coming as close to the floor as you can.

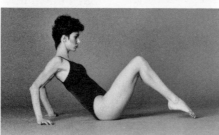

Come center.

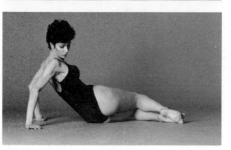

Then rotate your knees to the LEFT. Keep your stomach muscles in and your shoulders facing forward.

61
ADVANCED
HIP ROLLS
(30 SECONDS)

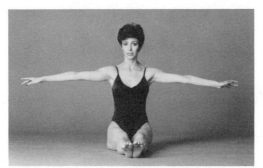

Sit with legs stretched out on the floor in front of you and arms out at shoulder height.

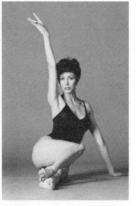
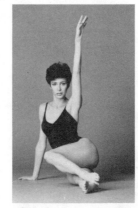

Swing RIGHT arm up over head as RIGHT hip comes off the floor.

Then swing LEFT arm over head as LEFT hip rolls off the floor. Swing directly to the side, keeping your body front.

62
BUTTOCKS LIFTS
(30 SECONDS)
(STRENGTHENS BUTTOCKS)

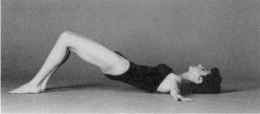

Lie on your back with your knees bent; feet parallel and hip distance apart on the floor; arms flat to the floor out to the side; stomach muscles in; pelvis raised off the floor. Raise and lower your pelvis in very small moves (only 4 inches up and down). Squeeze your buttocks muscles tight.

63
ADVANCED PELVICS
(30 SECONDS)

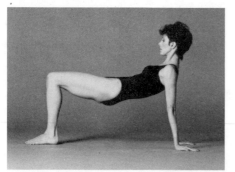

Support yourself on your hands, which are apart and behind you. Feet are parallel and flat on the floor. Knees are together and pelvis is raised off the floor 12 inches.

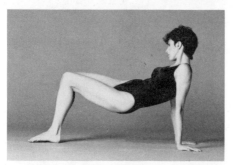

Swing your hips to the RIGHT. Come center.

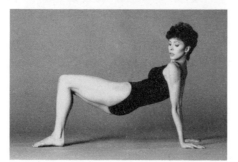

Then, swing your hips to the LEFT, keeping your stomach and buttocks muscles tight.

64
ULTRA PELVICS
(30 SECONDS)

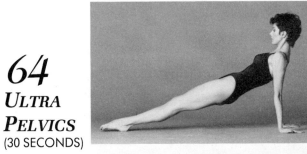

Support yourself on your hands, which are stretched out behind. Legs are stretched out long; toes are pointed and body is straight.

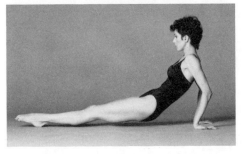

Lower pelvic area almost to the floor, bending your elbows. Then, raise up to starting position. Keep your stomach and buttocks muscles tight.

65
HIP RELEASE
(30 SECONDS)

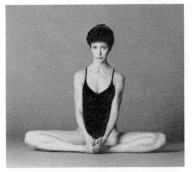

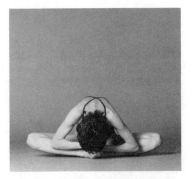

Sit up with the bottoms of your feet together and your back straight.

Round down over your legs, pressing your knees toward the floor. Hold for a count of 10. Then roll up.

SIDE LEGS WORKOUT

This workout was designed to tone and strengthen the muscles of your legs, hips, and thighs: specifically, the *gracilis* muscle on your inner thigh; the *pectineus*, or upper thigh muscle; the *adductor longus* muscle, located on the front of your upper thigh; the *quadriceps* of the outer thigh; and the *satorius*, the longest muscle in the body, which is also located on your inner thigh.

This routine also works on your abdominal and buttocks muscles.

Use the music listed for tone-ups in Chapter 7.

66

SIDE LEG LIFTS
(30 SECONDS)

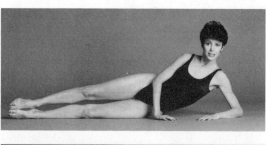

Lie on your LEFT hip, supporting your torso on your LEFT elbow and forearm; palms on the floor.

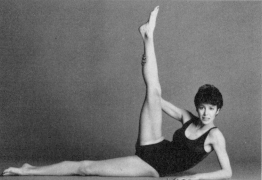

With toes pointed, lift your RIGHT leg up from the hip into a right angle with the floor and lower it, almost meeting the bottom leg. Stomach and buttocks tight. Lock that knee.

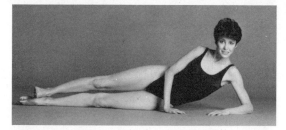

Then, with RIGHT foot flexed, raise RIGHT leg up and lower.

67
SCISSOR LEG LIFTS
(30 SECONDS)

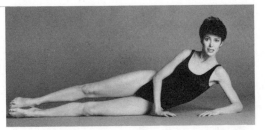

Lie on your LEFT hip, supporting your torso on your LEFT elbow; palms on the floor.

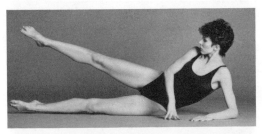

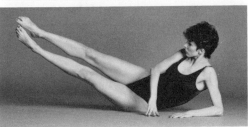

With toes pointed, bring RIGHT leg up in the air 12 inches.

Then, bring LEFT leg up to meet it. Keep RIGHT leg up in the air as you repeat the movement of the bottom leg. Don't let your body rock back.

68
V SCISSORS
(30 SECONDS)

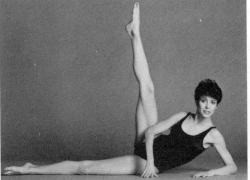

Lie on your LEFT hip, supporting your torso on your LEFT elbow; palms on the floor. Hold your RIGHT leg straight up as far as you can with RIGHT hand . . .

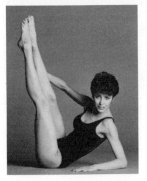

. . . bring LEFT leg up to meet it, then down to the floor. Continue to hold RIGHT leg in the air as you repeat the motion of the LEFT leg.

69
KNEE TO
FLOOR
(30 SECONDS)

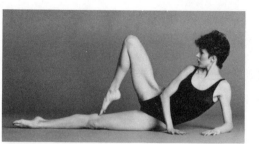

Lie on your LEFT hip, supporting your torso with your LEFT elbow; palms on the floor. Bend your RIGHT leg and place RIGHT foot on LEFT knee.

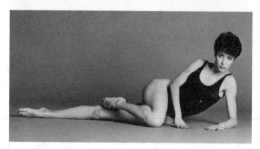

Swing RIGHT knee to floor and up to starting position. Keep your stomach muscles in and your body facing front. A down-and-up motion makes 1 count.

70
INNER
THIGH LIFT
(30 SECONDS)

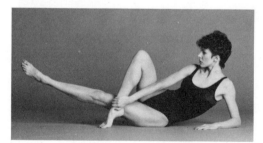

Lie on your LEFT side, supporting your torso on your LEFT elbow. Forearms and palms are flat on the floor. Lift your straight LEFT leg off the floor; toes are pointed; Grab your RIGHT foot with your RIGHT hand and put it in front of your LEFT leg. Lift and lower your LEFT leg in small moves. Keep your LEFT leg turned so that your inner thigh faces the ceiling.

Lie on your RIGHT side and repeat exercises #66 through #70 with your LEFT leg.

BUTTOCKS/THIGHS WORKOUT

This workout was designed to further help strengthen, firm, and tone the muscles of your buttocks and thighs: specifically, your *gluteus maximus*, *medius*, and *minimus*; *gracilis*; *pectineus*; and *adductor longus*. All of these muscles are very important in your ability to run and jump, two central aspects of aerobics.

Use the music listed for tone-ups in Chapter 7.

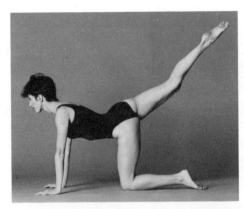

71
BACK LEG EXTENSIONS— RIGHT
(30 SECONDS)

Start on your hands and knees. Extend your RIGHT leg straight behind you with toes pointed. Using very small movements (6 inches up and down), raise and lower your leg. Don't throw it.

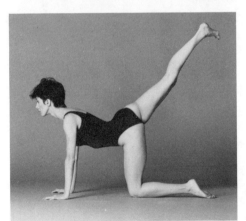

Then, with a flexed foot, continue the movement. Keep your back straight, your stomach muscles in, and your head up.

72
KNEE TO CHEST & OUT — RIGHT
(30 SECONDS)

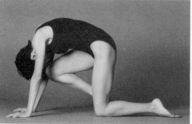

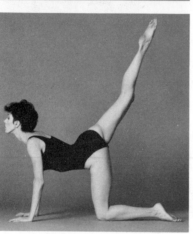

Start on your hands and knees. Bring your RIGHT knee in to your chest, contracting your back and bringing your head down.

Then, straighten your RIGHT leg back out while arching your body and raising your head. The 2 movements are done as 1 count in and out. Keep it a smooth, continuous motion.

73
SIDE LIFTS —RIGHT
(30 SECONDS)

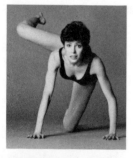

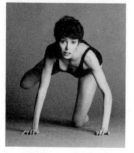

Start on your hands and knees. Lift bent RIGHT leg out to side at hip height, parallel to the ground.

Then, lower RIGHT leg almost to the floor. Keep your stomach muscles in and your hips still.

74
LEG SWINGS— RIGHT
(30 SECONDS)

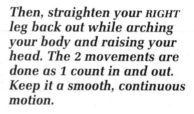

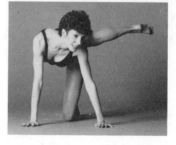

Start on your hands and knees. Raise your RIGHT leg out to the side in a swinging motion. Toes are pointed.

Then, swing it behind to the LEFT, crossing over your LEFT leg. A right-and-left motion makes 1 count. Repeat the motion. Keep it smooth.

75 HANDS & KNEES TRANSITION
(30 SECONDS)

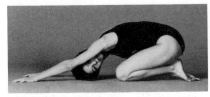

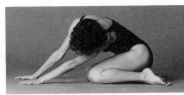

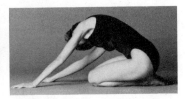

Sit back on your heels, then bend over with arms stretched out on the floor in front. Hold for 4 counts.

Then, hands still on the floor, sit over onto your RIGHT hip and hold.

Then, sit over onto LEFT hip and hold. This should relieve the tightness in your buttock muscles.

71
BACK LEG EXTENSIONS —LEFT
(30 SECONDS)

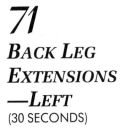

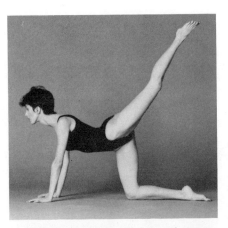

Start on your hands and knees. Extend your LEFT leg straight behind you with toes pointed. Using very small movements (6 inches up and down), raise and lower your leg.

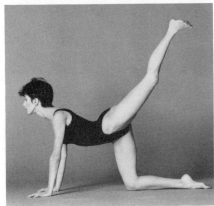

Then, with a flexed foot, continue the movement.

72
KNEE TO CHEST & OUT— LEFT
(30 SECONDS)

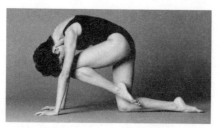

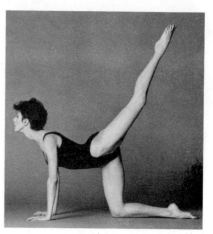

Bring your LEFT knee in to your chest, contracting your back and bringing your head down.

Then, straighten your LEFT leg back out while arching your body and raising your head.

73
SIDE LIFTS —LEFT
(30 SECONDS)

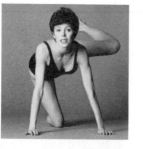

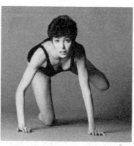

Start on your hands and knees. Lift bent LEFT leg out to side at hip level, parallel to the ground.

Lower your leg almost to the floor. Keep your stomach muscles in and your hips still.

74
LEG SWINGS —LEFT
(30 SECONDS)

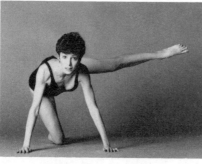

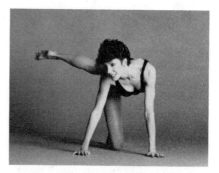

Start on your hands and knees. Raise your LEFT leg straight out to the side in a swinging motion. Toes are pointed.

Then, swing LEFT leg behind to the RIGHT, crossing over your RIGHT leg. A left-and-right motion makes 1 count. Repeat the motion. Keep it smooth.

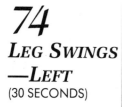
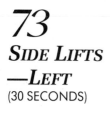

76
THIGH TILT BACK
(30 SECONDS)

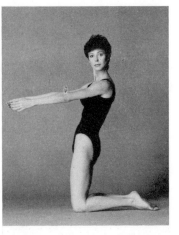 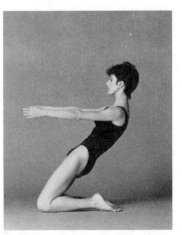

Kneel on the floor with legs together; stomach in; hips tucked under; arms out straight to the front.

Keeping your body in a straight line, arms extended, tilt back toward your heels; hold for a count of 10; and come up straight. Keep your back straight and stomach muscles in.

75
HANDS & KNEES TRANSITION
(30 SECONDS)

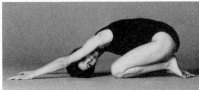 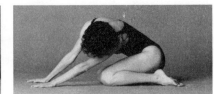 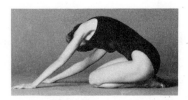

Sit back on your heels, then bend over with arms stretched out on the floor in front. Hold for 4 counts.

Then, hands still on the floor, sit over onto RIGHT hip and hold.

Then, sit over onto LEFT hip and hold.

CHAPTER SEVEN

LOUD MUSIC

Music quickens time, she quickens us to the finest enjoyment of time.

—Thomas Mann (1924)

Music is the key to our Aerobicise program. Without it your workout pace would slow down and then speed up and then slow down again. You would be on a roller coaster and be unable to get the effects of *sustained* aerobic conditioning that you want. Since most other aerobic sports are done without the beat of music, it's easy to slack off during an exercise routine. That prohibits you from consistently moving fast enough to complete your workout in just 12 minutes.

The Louder the Music, the More Energy It Will Give You

Music acts as a coach, urging you to keep going. The louder and faster the music, the more you are inspired to keep up with its beat.

Anyone who has ever gone dancing can tell you how much fun it is and how much energy music seems to give you. This is precisely why our Aerobicise program works: Exercise done to music is easier and more fun to do, so you keep at it without slowing your pace.

Recent research by Jane Standley, Ph.D., director of music therapy at Florida State University in Tallahassee, on the physical and psychological effects of music on human beings substantiates this. She has found that listening to soothing music can slow the pulse and relax us, while hearing a fast beat can increase pulse rate, energize people, and make them want to get up and move around.[1]

And in a controlled experiment at Ohio State University in Columbus, runners who listened to upbeat music perceived themselves to be experiencing considerably less physical stress than runners who were not listening to music, even though both groups were actually expending the same amount of energy.

There are at least two theories to explain the Ohio State phenomenon: The runners were able to concentrate on the music rather than on the task of exercising; and the music activated a release of endorphins, which gave the runners a "natural high" and raised their tolerance for physical discomfort. (Music seems to be so successful in masking pain and inspiring great physical feats that it is now used in conjunction with Lamaze breathing techniques in many delivery rooms.)[2]

To test my belief that loud, fast music is the critical difference between our Aerobicise program and all the other aerobic sports, I went to Santa Monica, where a large concentration of weekend joggers in Southern California gathers. I brought my stopwatch with me and timed several hundred joggers to see what their average speed was.

What I had suspected I now know to be true. The joggers averaged moving at 95 steps, or beats, per minute. Now if those joggers were out of shape, they were getting their heartbeat into their target zones, but if they were in decent shape, they were probably getting little or no cardiovascular benefit from jogging so slowly.

If you are in shape and you are jogging at 95 beats per minute, it will take you approximately 45 minutes to do what you could in 12 minutes with Aerobicise and music that has 120 beats per minute.

This chapter lists the top 400 popular songs that are the best for our Aerobicise routines. Each song is listed with the beats per minute (BPM) noted alongside. If you wish to slow down or speed up your workouts, just choose a song with different beats per minute.

The songs are also broken down into workout segment (Warm-Ups, Aerobics, Cool-Downs, Tone-Ups) and body part they will benefit. Please note that songs recommended for Tone-Ups, Warm-Ups, and Cool-Downs can be adapted to any of those three activities. If you find that you like a particular song better for one of the three segments other than our recommendation, go ahead and use it. We have listed those songs according to their primary use only. This does not apply to the Aerobics songs. They have been chosen specifically for their fast beat and should be used exclusively for the Aerobics portion of your workout.

Also, you may find that even though the beats per minute are the same on two songs, the sound of the songs may be different enough to make you feel that one is more appropriate for warming up, while the other seems better suited to cooling down. Follow your own body's perceptions in choosing music for your workout.

We've included current songs and some from the recent past. We hope you will have some of them in your record collection.

If you're a beginner, we recommend you start with music that has slower beats per minute. The following chart contains a list of beats per minute to guide the beginner, the intermediate, or the advanced participant. The chart also corresponds to the workouts you will find in Chapter 5.

Play the music as loud as you and your neighbors can stand it; the louder the music, the more you will be able to do. To be considerate, you might want to consider buying a Sony Walkman (the smallest Walkman has a strap and belt hook to keep it from swinging while you jump). You can get one for around $75 at your local discount store. With a Walkman, you can play the music as loud as you like without disturbing anyone.

BEATS PER MINUTE

	WARM-UP	AEROBICS	COOL-DOWN
VERY OUT OF SHAPE	96	108	96
OUT OF SHAPE	102	114	102
GETTING IN SHAPE	108	120	108
IN SHAPE	114	126	114
GREAT SHAPE	120	132	120
FABULOUS SHAPE	126	138	126
IN TRAINING	132	144	132

MUSIC IN BEATS PER MINUTE FOR AEROBICISE

SONG	ARTIST	ALBUM	REC. CO.	NUMBER	BODY/ONE*	BODY/TWO**	SEGMENT	BPM
Mornin'	Al Jarreau	Jarreau	WB	23801-1	Legs	Back	Cool-Down	96
Here She Comes	Bonnie Tyler	Metropolis	Columbia	JS-39526	Legs	Back	Cool-Down	96
One on One	Hall & Oates	H$_2$O	RCA	ALF1-4383	Legs	Back	Cool-Down	102
The Safety Dance	Men Without Hats	Rhythm of Youth	Backstreet	BSR-39002	Legs	Back	Cool-Down	102
Simple Things	Minnie Riperton	Adventures in Paradise	Epic	PE-33454	Legs	Back	Cool-Down	102
Superstition	Stevie Wonder	Talking Book	Motown	T-319L	Legs	Back	Cool-Down	102
Hot Stuff	The Rolling Stones	Black & Blue	Roln'Stons	COC-79104	Legs	Back	Cool-Down	102
Human Nature	Michael Jackson	Thriller	Epic	QE-38112	Waist	Back	Cool-Down	102
Spinning	Christopher Cross	Christopher Cross	WB	BSK-3383	Back	Legs	Cool-Down	108
New Kid in Town	Eagles	Hotel California	Asylum	7E-1084	Back	Legs	Cool-Down	108
I Can't Help It	Michael Jackson	Off the Wall	Epic	FE-35745	Back	Legs	Cool-Down	108
Ain't Nobody	Rufus & Chaka Khan	Stomping at the Savoy	WB	923679-1	Back	Legs	Cool-Down	108
Sweet Somebody	Shannon	Let the Music Play	Mirage	90134-1	Back	Legs	Cool-Down	108
How Deep Is Your Love	Bee Gees	Saturday Night Fever	RSO	RS-24001	Legs	Back	Cool-Down	108
More Than a Woman	Bee Gees	Saturday Night Fever	RSO	RS-24001	Legs	Back	Cool-Down	108
Stayin' Alive	Bee Gees	Saturday Night Fever	RSO	RS-24001	Legs	Back	Cool-Down	108
Loverboy	Billy Ocean	Suddenly	Arista	JL-88213	Legs	Back	Cool-Down	108
You're So Vain	Carly Simon	No Secrets	Elektra	75045	Legs	Back	Cool-Down	108
Feels So Good	Chuck Mangione	Feels So Good	A&M	SP-4697	Legs	Back	Cool-Down	108
Winter Melody	Donna Summer	Four Seasons of Love	Casablanca	NBLP-7038	Legs	Back	Cool-Down	108
Love to Love You Baby	Donna Summer	Love to Love You Baby	Casablanca	OCLP-5003	Legs	Back	Cool-Down	108
Yearnin' Learnin'	Earth, Wind and Fire	The Way of the World	Columbia	PC-33280	Legs	Back	Cool-Down	108
Shining Star	Earth, Wind and Fire	The Way of the World	Columbia	PC-33280	Legs	Back	Cool-Down	108
Affirmation	George Benson	Breezin'	WB	0698	Legs	Back	Cool-Down	108
Red Hot	Herb Alpert	Blow Your Own Horn	A&M	SP-4949	Legs	Back	Cool-Down	108

* The primary body area for which this song is good.
** The secondary body area for which this song is good.

	ARTIST	ALBUM	REC. CO.	NUMBER	BODY/ONE*	BODY/TWO**	SEGMENT	BPM
Chameleon	Herbie Hancock	Headhunters	Columbia	PC-32721	Legs	Back	Cool-Down	108
Steppin' In It	Herbie Hancock	Man-Child	Columbia	PC-33812	Legs	Back	Cool-Down	108
If This Is It	Huey Lewis and the News	Sports	Chrysalis	FV-41412	Legs	Back	Cool-Down	108
Is It Right	Jeffrey Osborne	Don't Stop	A&M	SP-5017	Legs	Back	Cool-Down	108
You Can't Be Serious	Jeffrey Osborne	Don't Stop	A&M	SP-5017	Legs	Back	Cool-Down	108
Do What You Do	Jermaine Jackson	Jermaine Jackson	Arista	AL-88203	Legs	Back	Cool-Down	108
Tell Me I'm Not Dreamin'	Jermaine Jackson	Jermaine Jackson	Arista	AL-88203	Legs	Back	Cool-Down	108
This Is It	Kenny Loggins	Keep the Fire	Columbia	JC-36172	Legs	Back	Cool-Down	108
Down Under	Men at Work	Business as Usual	Columbia	FC-37978	Legs	Back	Cool-Down	108
Baby Be Mine	Michael Jackson	Thriller	Epic	QE-38112	Legs	Back	Cool-Down	108
Adventures in Paradise	Minnie Riperton	Adventures in Paradise	Epic	PE-33454	Legs	Back	Cool-Down	108
DMSR	Prince	Prince 1999	WB	23720-F	Legs	Back	Cool-Down	108
True	Spandau Ballet	True	Chrysalis	FV-41403	Legs	Back	Cool-Down	108
On and On	Stephen Bishop	Careless	ABC	ABCD-954	Legs	Back	Cool-Down	108
Crazy	Supertramp	Famous Last Words	A&M	SP-3732	Legs	Back	Cool-Down	108
Playboy	Teena Marie	Robbery	Epic	FE-38882	Legs	Back	Cool-Down	108
Listen to the Music	The Doobie Brothers	Best of the Doobies	WB	BS-2978	Legs	Back	Cool-Down	108
Just Be Good to Me	The SOS Band	On the Rise	Tabu	F238697	Legs	Back	Cool-Down	108
Let's Stay Together	Tina Turner	Private Dancer	EMI	ST-12330	Legs	Back	Cool-Down	108
What's Love Got to Do With It	Tina Turner	Private Dancer	EMI	ST-12330	Legs	Back	Cool-Down	108
If I Can't Have You	Yvonne Elliman	Saturday Night Fever	RSO	RS-24001	Legs	Back	Cool-Down	108
Somethin' Special	Quincy Jones	The Dude	A&M	SP-3721	Legs	Waist	Cool-Down	108
The Power	Jeffrey Osborne	Don't Stop	A&M	SP-5017	Waist	Legs	Cool-Down	108

Song	Artist	Label	Album	Catalog				
Lie to Me	Depeche Mode	Sire	Some Great Reward	25194-1	Back	Legs	Cool-Down	114
Do Ya Think I'm Sexy	Rod Stewart	WB	Blondes Have More Fun	BSX-3261	Back	Legs	Cool-Down	114
Relax	Frankie Goes to Hollywood	Island	LP Single	0-96975	Back	Waist	Cool-Down	114
Boogie Down	Al Jarreau	WB	Jarreau	23801-1	Legs	Back	Cool-Down	114
Step by Step	Al Jarreau	WB	Jarreau	23801-1	Legs	Back	Cool-Down	114
Night Fever	Bee Gees	RSO	Saturday Night Fever	RS-24001	Legs	Back	Cool-Down	114
Jive Talkin'	Bee Gees	RSO	Saturday Night Fever	RS-24001	Legs	Back	Cool-Down	114
Waited So Long	Carly Simon	Elektra	No Secrets	75045	Legs	Back	Cool-Down	114
Chic Cheer	Chic	Atlantic	Chic's Greatest Hits	SD-16011	Legs	Back	Cool-Down	114
Good Times	Chic	Atlantic	Chic's Greatest Hits	SD-16011	Legs	Back	Cool-Down	114
Autumn Changes	Donna Summer	Casablanca	Four Seasons of Love	NBLP-7038	Legs	Back	Cool-Down	114
If You Got It Flaunt It	Donna Summer	Casablanca	Once Upon a Time	NBLP-7078	Legs	Back	Cool-Down	114
Life in the Fast Lane	Eagles	Asylum	Hotel California	7E-1084	Legs	Back	Cool-Down	114
Jeopardy	Greg Kihnspiracy Band	Beserkley	LP Single	0-67932	Legs	Back	Cool-Down	114
I Can't Go for That	Hall & Oates	RCA	Rock 'n Soul, Part 1	CPL1-4858	Legs	Back	Cool-Down	114
Autodrive	Herbie Hancock	Columbia	Future Shock	FC-38814	Legs	Back	Cool-Down	114
Rockit	Herbie Hancock	Columbia	Future Shock	FC-38814	Legs	Back	Cool-Down	114
Come to Me	Jermaine Jackson	Arista	Jermaine Jackson	AL-88203	Legs	Back	Cool-Down	114
Keep the Fire	Kenny Loggins	Columbia	Keep the Fire	JC-36172	Legs	Back	Cool-Down	114
Don't Want to Live Without It	Pablo Cruise	A&M	Worlds Away	SP-4697	Legs	Back	Cool-Down	114
A Fifth of Beethoven	Walter Murphy	RSO	Saturday Night Fever	RS-24001	Legs	Back	Cool-Down	114
Poor Shirley	Christopher Cross	WB	Christopher Cross	BSK-3383	Legs	Buttocks	Cool-Down	114
Something Like a Dream	Vicki Sue Robinson	RCA	Vicki Sue Robinson	APL1-1829	Legs	Waist	Cool-Down	114
Thriller	Michael Jackson	Epic	Thriller	QE-38112	Back	Buttocks	Cool-Down	120
All the Things Are Nice	General Public	IRS	All the Rage	SP-70046	Back	Legs	Cool-Down	120

* The primary body area for which this song is good.
** The secondary body area for which this song is good.

	ARTIST	ALBUM	REC. CO.	NUMBER	BODY/ONE*	BODY/TWO**	SEGMENT	BPM
Out of Touch	Hall & Oates	Big Bam Boom	RCA	AFL1-5309	Back	Legs	Cool-Down	120
Lucky Star	Madonna	Madonna	Sire	1-23867	Back	Legs	Cool-Down	120
Rock With You	Michael Jackson	Off the Wall	Epic	FE-35745	Back	Legs	Cool-Down	120
Billy Jean	Michael Jackson	Thriller	Epic	QE-38112	Back	Legs	Cool-Down	120
Black & Blues	Al Jarreau	Jarreau	WB	23801-1	Legs	Back	Cool-Down	120
Need a Man Blues	Bronski Beat	The Age of Consent	MCA	MCA-5538	Legs	Back	Cool-Down	120
We Have No Secrets	Carly Simon	No Secrets	Elektra	75045	Legs	Back	Cool-Down	120
I Want Your Love	Chic	Chic's Greatest Hits	Atlantic	SD-16011	Legs	Back	Cool-Down	120
Hide and Seek	Chuck Mangione	Feels So Good	A&M	SP-4658	Legs	Back	Cool-Down	120
Country Girl	Crosby, Stills, Nash & Young	Déjà Vu	Atlantic	SD-7200	Legs	Back	Cool-Down	120
It's a Miracle	Culture Club	Color by Numbers	Epic	QE-39107	Legs	Back	Cool-Down	120
Swept Away	Diana Ross	Swept Away	RCA	AFL-15009	Legs	Back	Cool-Down	120
Save a Prayer	Duran Duran	Arena	EMI	SWAV-12374	Legs	Back	Cool-Down	120
Reasons	Earth, Wind and Fire	The Way of the World	Columbia	PC-33280	Legs	Back	Cool-Down	120
Cry Now, Laugh Later	Grace Jones	Living My Life	Island	90018-1	Legs	Back	Cool-Down	120
Say It Isn't So	Hall & Oates	Rock 'n Soul, Part 1	RCA	CPL1-4858	Legs	Back	Cool-Down	120
The Traitor	Herbie Hancock	Man-Child	Columbia	PC-33812	Legs	Back	Cool-Down	120
Better Be Good to Me	Tina Turner	Private Dancer	EMI	ST-12330	Legs	Buttocks	Cool-Down	120
Rain Forest	Paul Hardcastle	LP Single	Profile	7059	Waist	Back	Cool-Down	120
Sex Shooter	Apollonia Six	Apollonia 6	WB	1-25108	Buttocks	Waist	Tone-Up	120
Machines	Giorgio Moroder	Metropolis	Columbia	JS-39526	Stomach	Arms	Tone-Up	120
Der Kommissar	Falco	Einzeilhaft	A&M	SP-64951	Stomach	Buttocks	Tone-Up	120
Jungle Love	The Time	Ice Cream Castles	WB	25109-1	Stomach	Legs	Tone-Up	120
State of Shock	M. Jackson/M. Jagger	Victory	Epic	QE-38946	Stomach	Waist	Tone-Up	120
Summer Love	Musique	Keep On Jumpin'	Prelude	PRL-12158	Arms	Legs	Warm-Up	120
Off the Wall	Michael Jackson	Off the Wall	Epic	FE-35745	Arms	Stomach	Warm-Up	120
Money Changes Everything	Cyndi Lauper	She's So Unusual	Portrait	FR-38930	Arms	Waist	Warm-Up	120

Song	Artist	Album	Label	Catalog No.	Body Area*	Body Area**	Section	BPM
Calypso Breakdown	Ralph McDonald	Saturday Night Fever	RSO	RS-24001	Arms	Waist	Warm-Up	120
Day Light	Vicki Sue Robinson	Vicki Sue Robinson	RCA	APL1-1829	Legs	Waist	Warm-Up	120
Heart of Glass	Blondie	Parallel Lines	Chrysalis	CHR-1192	Waist	Arms	Warm-Up	120
Hang Up Your Hang-Ups	Herbie Hancock	Man-Child	Columbia	PC-33812	Waist	Arms	Warm-Up	120
Open Sesame	Kool and the Gang	Saturday Night Fever	RSO	RS-24001	Waist	Arms	Warm-Up	120
I Wanna Be Your Lover	Prince	Prince	WB	BSK-3366	Waist	Arms	Warm-Up	120
The Politics of Dancing	RE-Flex	The Politics of Dancing	Capital	ST-12314	Waist	Arms	Warm-Up	120
Physical Attraction	Madonna	LP Single	Sire	9-29715	Waist	Back	Warm-Up	120
Woodstock	Crosby, Stills, Nash & Young	Déjà Vu	Atlantic	SD-7200	Waist	Buttocks	Warm-Up	120
Wild Boys	Duran Duran	Arena	EMI	SWAV-12374	Waist	Buttocks	Warm-Up	120
Unison	Junior	LP Single	Casablanca	814-7251	Waist	Buttocks	Warm-Up	120
Le Freak	Chic	Chic's Greatest Hits	Atlantic	SD-16011	Waist	Legs	Warm-Up	120
Sweet Dynamite	Claudja Barry	Sweet Dynamite	Salsoul	SZS-5512	Waist	Legs	Warm-Up	120
I'll Tumble 4 Ya	Culture Club	LP Single	Virgin	VS612	Waist	Legs	Warm-Up	120
Queen for a Day	Donna Summer	Once Upon a Time	Casablanca	NBLP-7078	Waist	Legs	Warm-Up	120
The Day Before You Came	General Public	All the Rage	IRS	SP-70046	Waist	Legs	Warm-Up	120
Unlimited Capacity for Love	Grace Jones	Living My Life	Island	90018-1	Waist	Legs	Warm-Up	120
Borderline	Madonna	Madonna	Sire	1-23867	Waist	Legs	Warm-Up	120
Let the Music Play	Shannon	Let the Music Play	Mirage	90134-1	Waist	Legs	Warm-Up	120
Give Me Tonight	Shannon	Let the Music Play	Mirage	90134-1	Waist	Legs	Warm-Up	120
My Heart's Divided	Shannon	Let the Music Play	Mirage	90134-1	Waist	Legs	Warm-Up	120
Long Train Runnin'	The Doobie Brothers	Best of the Doobies	WB	BS-2978	Waist	Legs	Warm-Up	120
Caribbean Queen	Billy Ocean	LP Single	Jive	JDI-9215	Waist	Stomach	Warm-Up	120
Heart and Soul	Huey Lewis and the News	Sports	Chrysalis	FV-41412	Waist	Stomach	Warm-Up	120
I'll Kiss You	Cyndi Lauper	She's So Unusual	Portrait	FR-38930	Heart	Stomach	Aerobics	126

* The primary body area for which this song is good.
** The secondary body area for which this song is good.

ARTIST	ALBUM	REC. CO.	NUMBER	BODY/ONE*	BODY/TWO**	SEGMENT	BPM
The Time	Ice Cream Castles	WB	25109-1	Heart	Stomach	Aerobics	126
Christopher Cross	Christopher Cross	WB	BSK-3383	Stomach	Legs	Aerobics	126
Donna Summer	A Love Trilogy	Oasis	OCLP-5004	Arms	Legs	Cool-Down	126
Cyndi Lauper	She's So Unusual	Portrait	FR-38930	Back	Legs	Cool-Down	126
Carly Simon	Hello Big Man	WB	23886-1	Legs	Back	Cool-Down	126
Christopher Cross	Christopher Cross	WB	BSK-3383	Legs	Back	Cool-Down	126
Donna Summer	Four Seasons of Love	Casablanca	NBLP-7038	Legs	Back	Cool-Down	126
Fleetwood Mac	Rumours	WB	BSK-3010	Legs	Back	Cool-Down	126
General Public	All the Rage	IRS	SP-70046	Legs	Back	Cool-Down	126
Gino Soccio	Outline	RFC/WB	RFC-3309	Legs	Back	Cool-Down	126
Grace Jones	Living My Life	Island	90018-1	Legs	Back	Cool-Down	126
Olivia Newton-John	Never Been Mellow	MCA	2133	Legs	Back	Cool-Down	126
Prince and The Revolution	Purple Rain	WB	26110-1	Legs	Back	Cool-Down	126
Shandi	Flashdance	Casablanca	811492	Legs	Back	Cool-Down	126
Karla Bonoff	Footloose	Columbia	JS-39242	Legs	Waist	Cool-Down	126
Olivia Newton-John	Never Been Mellow	MCA	2133	Legs	Waist	Cool-Down	126
Rod Stewart	Blondes Have More Fun	WB	BSK-3261	Legs	Waist	Cool-Down	126
Shalimar	Footloose	Columbia	JS-39242	Stomach	Buttocks	Cool-Down	126
Michael Jackson	Off the Wall	Epic	FE-35745	Waist	Arms	Cool-Down	126
Giorgio Moroder	Midnight Express	Casablanca	NBLP-7114	Buttocks	Stomach	Tone-Up	126
Laid Back	White Horse	Sire	20178-0-A	Buttocks	Stomach	Tone-Up	126
Rockwell	Somebody's Watching Me	Motown	6052-ML	Buttocks	Stomach	Tone-Up	126
Temper	LP Single	MCA	MCA-23506	Buttocks	Stomach	Tone-Up	126
Devine	LP Single	Break	308327	Buttocks	Waist	Tone-Up	126
Bee Gees	Saturday Night Fever	RSO	RS2-4001	Stomach	Buttocks	Tone-Up	126
Carly Simon	No Secrets	Elektra	75045	Stomach	Buttocks	Tone-Up	126
Cerrone	Supernature	Cotillion	SD-5202	Stomach	Buttocks	Tone-Up	126
MFSB	Saturday Night Fever	RSO	RS-24001	Stomach	Buttocks	Tone-Up	126

Song titles (first column):
The Bird; Ride Like the Wind; Try Me, I Know We Can Make It; Time After Time; Hello Big Man; The Light Is On; Summer Fever; Gold Dust Woman; Don't Tell Me; Dancer; Inspiration; Goodbye Again; Take Me With You; He's a Dream; Somebody's Eyes; Follow Me; Ain't Love a Bitch; Dancing in the Streets; Don't Stop 'Til You Get Enough; Chase; White Horse; Somebody's Watching Me; No Favors; Love Reaction; You Should Be Dancing; Night Owl; Supernature; K-Jee

Song	Artist	Album	Label	Catalog				
Fix It	Teena Marie	Robbery	Epic	FE-38882	Stomach	Buttocks	Tone-Up	126
Lovergirl	Teena Marie	Star Child	Epic	FE-39528	Stomach	Buttocks	Tone-Up	126
Love Will Find a Way	Pablo Cruise	Worlds Away	A&M	SP-4697	Stomach	Waist	Tone-Up	126
Dance to Dance	Gino Soccio	Outline	RFC/WB	RFC-3309	Waist	Legs	Tone-Up	126
Menergy	Patrick Cowley	LP Single	Megatone	NONE	Waist	Legs	Tone-Up	126
Cerrone's Paradise	Cerrone	Cerrone's Paradise	Cotillion	SD-9917	Waist	Stomach	Tone-Up	126
When You Were Mine	Cyndi Lauper	She's So Unusual	Portrait	FR-38930	Arms	Buttocks	Warm-Up	126
You're My Magician	Lime	Your Love	Prism	PLP-1008	Arms	Buttocks	Warm-Up	126
Girls Just Want to Have Fun	Cyndi Lauper	She's So Unusual	Portrait	FR-38930	Arms	Legs	Warm-Up	126
It's Raining Again	Supertramp	Famous Last Words	A&M	SP-3732	Arms	Legs	Warm-Up	126
I Really Don't Know Anymore	Christopher Cross	Christopher Cross	WB	BSK-3383	Arms	Waist	Warm-Up	126
Never Be the Same	Christopher Cross	Christopher Cross	WB	BSK-3383	Arms	Waist	Warm-Up	126
Take Me	Donna Summer	I Remember Yesterday	Casablanca	NBLP-7056	Arms	Waist	Warm-Up	126
Too Hot to Handle	Giorgio	From Here to Eternity	Casablanca	NBLP-7065	Arms	Waist	Warm-Up	126
TFS	Herbie Hancock	Future Shock	Columbia	FC-38814	Arms	Waist	Warm-Up	126
I Love You So	Manny's	LP Single	DJ Records	DJD-019	Arms	Waist	Warm-Up	126
Family Man	Pablo Cruise	Worlds Away	A&M	SP-4697	Stomach	Buttocks	Warm-Up	126
20th Century Foxes	Angel	Foxes	Casablanca	NBLP-27206	Waist	Arms	Warm-Up	126
I Feel for You	Chaka Khan	I Feel for You	WB	25162-1	Waist	Arms	Warm-Up	126
Dance, Dance, Dance	Chic	Chic's Greatest Hits	Atlantic	SD-16011	Waist	Arms	Warm-Up	126
Miss Me Blind	Culture Club	Color by Numbers	Epic	QE-39107	Waist	Arms	Warm-Up	126
Manhattan Sky Line	David Shire	Saturday Night Fever	RSO	RS-24001	Waist	Arms	Warm-Up	126
Let's Hear It for the Boy	Deniece Williams	Footloose	Columbia	JS-39242	Waist	Arms	Warm-Up	126
Salsation	David Shire	Saturday Night Fever	RSO	RS-24001	Waist	Arms	Warm-Up	126
Working the Midnight Shift	Donna Summer	Once Upon a Time	Casablanca	NBLP-7078	Waist	Arms	Warm-Up	126
Now I Need You	Donna Summer	Once Upon a Time	Casablanca	NBLP-7078	Waist	Arms	Warm-Up	126
Dreams	Fleetwood Mac	Rumours	WB	BSK-3010	Waist	Arms	Warm-Up	126
On Broadway	George Benson	All That Jazz	Casablanca	NBLP-7198	Waist	Arms	Warm-Up	126
Utopia	Giorgio	From Here to Eternity	Casablanca	NBLP-7065	Waist	Arms	Warm-Up	126
1st Hand Experience in 2nd Hand Love	Giorgio	From Here to Eternity	Casablanca	NBLP-7065	Waist	Arms	Warm-Up	126

* The primary body area for which this song is good.
** The secondary body area for which this song is good.

Song	ARTIST	ALBUM	REC. CO.	NUMBER	BODY/ONE*	BODY/TWO**	SEGMENT	BPM
Kiss on My List	Hall & Oates	Rock'n Soul, Part 1	RCA	CPL1-4858	Waist	Arms	Warm-Up	126
What a Feeling	Irene Cara	Flashdance	Casablanca	811492	Waist	Arms	Warm-Up	126
Wanna Be Startin' Something	Michael Jackson	Thriller	Epic	QE-38112	Waist	Arms	Warm-Up	126
Sexy Dancer	Prince	Prince	WB	BSK-3366	Waist	Arms	Warm-Up	126
Little Red Corvette	Prince	Prince 1999	WB	23720-F	Waist	Arms	Warm-Up	126
How About Me	Vicki Sue Robinson	Vicki Sue Robinson	RCA	APLP-1829	Waist	Arms	Warm-Up	126
Should I Stay	Vicki Sue Robinson	Vicki Sue Robinson	RCA	APL1-1829	Waist	Arms	Warm-Up	126
Have You Never Been Mellow	Olivia Newton-John	Never Been Mellow	MCA	2133	Waist	Legs	Warm-Up	126
Megamelody	Patrick Cowley	LP Single	Megatone	NONE	Waist	Legs	Warm-Up	126
Mange Tout	Blanc Mange	Mange Tout	Sire	25172-1	Waist	Stomach	Warm-Up	126
Blind Vision	General Public	All the Rage	IRS	SP-70046	Waist	Stomach	Warm-Up	126
Private Eyes	Hall & Oates	Rock'n Soul, Part 1	RCA	CPL1-4858	Waist	Stomach	Warm-Up	126
1999	Prince	Prince 1999	WB	23720-F	Waist	Stomach	Warm-Up	126
When Doves Cry	Prince and The Revolution	Purple Rain	WB	26110-1	Waist	Stomach	Warm-Up	126
Razzamatazz	Quincy Jones	The Dude	A&M	SP-3721	Waist	Stomach	Warm-Up	126
Spring Affair	Donna Summer	Four Seasons of Love	Casablanca	NBLP-7038	Arms	Stomach	Warm-Up	126
Midnight Lady	Cerrone	Love in C Minor	Cotillion	SD-9913	Heart	Buttocks	Aerobics	132
I Remember Yesterday	Donna Summer	I Remember Yesterday	Casablanca	NBLP-7056	Heart	Buttocks	Aerobics	132
Fairy Tale High	Donna Summer	Once Upon a Time	Casablanca	NBLP-7078	Heart	Buttocks	Aerobics	132
Once Upon a Time	Donna Summer	Once Upon a Time	Casablanca	NBLP-7078	Heart	Buttocks	Aerobics	132
Let Go	France Joli	France Joli	Prelude	12170-0798	Heart	Buttocks	Aerobics	132
Superman	Herbie Mann	Superman	Atlantic	SD-19221	Heart	Buttocks	Aerobics	132
Agent 406	Lime	Your Love	Prism	PLP-1008	Heart	Buttocks	Aerobics	132
In the Bush	Musique	Keep On Jumpin'	Prelude	PRL-12158	Heart	Buttocks	Aerobics	132
Again and Again	Nikki Lauren	LP Single	Wave	DL-1218	Heart	Buttocks	Aerobics	132
Shake It	Brooklyn Dreams	Foxes	Casablanca	NBLP-27206	Heart	Legs	Aerobics	132
Give Me Love	Cerrone	Supernature	Cotillion	SD-5202	Heart	Legs	Aerobics	132
I Feel Love (Original)	Donna Summer	I Remember Yesterday	Casablanca	NBLP-7056	Heart	Legs	Aerobics	132
Rumor Has It	Donna Summer	Once Upon a Time	Casablanca	NBLP-7078	Heart	Legs	Aerobics	132
From Here to Eternity	Giorgio	From Here to Eternity	Casablanca	SD-9913	Heart	Legs	Aerobics	132

Song	Artist	Album	Label	Catalog				
Jisco Dazz	Herbie Mann	Superman	Atlantic	SD-19221	Heart	Legs	Aerobics	132
Jump	Van Halen	1984	WB	923985-1	Heart	Legs	Aerobics	132
Scotch Machine	Voyage	Voyage	Marlin	2213	Heart	Legs	Aerobics	132
Smalltown Boy	Bronski Beat	The Age of Consent	MCA	MCA-5538	Heart	Stomach	Aerobics	132
Junk	Bronski Beat	The Age of Consent	MCA	MCA-5538	Heart	Stomach	Aerobics	132
Happiness Pill	Cerrone	Cerrone 6—Panic	Malligator	UPLP-19	Heart	Stomach	Aerobics	132
Love in C Minor	Cerrone	Love in C Minor	Cotillion	SD-9913	Heart	Stomach	Aerobics	132
Love Is the Answer	Cerrone	Supernature	Cotillion	SD-5202	Heart	Stomach	Aerobics	132
Badlove	Cher/Giorgio Moroder	Foxes	Casablanca	NBLP-27206	Heart	Stomach	Aerobics	132
Everybody Dance	Chic	Chic's Greatest Hits	Atlantic	SD-16011	Heart	Stomach	Aerobics	132
Church of the Poison Mind	Culture Club	Color by Numbers	Epic	QE-39107	Heart	Stomach	Aerobics	132
Master and Servant	Depeche Mode	Some Great Reward	Sire	25194-1	Heart	Stomach	Aerobics	132
Happily Ever After	Donna Summer	Once Upon a Time	Casablanca	NBLP-7078	Heart	Stomach	Aerobics	132
Faster & Faster to Nowhere	Donna Summer	Once Upon a Time	Casablanca	NBLP-7078	Heart	Stomach	Aerobics	132
Africano	Earth, Wind and Fire	The Way of the World	Columbia	PC-33280	Heart	Stomach	Aerobics	132
Don't Go Breaking My Heart	Elton John	Greatest Hits #2	MCA	3027	Heart	Stomach	Aerobics	132
Don't Stop Dancing	France Joli	France Joli	Prelude	12170-0798	Heart	Stomach	Aerobics	132
Two Tribes	Frankie Goes to Hollywood	LP Single	Island	0-96931	Heart	Stomach	Aerobics	132
Valley of the Dolls	Giorgio Moroder	Foxes	Casablanca	NBLP-27206	Heart	Stomach	Aerobics	132
Rock Freak	Herbie Mann	Superman	Atlantic	SD-19221	Heart	Stomach	Aerobics	132
Stamp Your Feet	Herbie Mann	Superman	Atlantic	SD-19221	Heart	Stomach	Aerobics	132
Body Oil	Herbie Mann	Superman	Atlantic	SD-19221	Heart	Stomach	Aerobics	132
The Borderline	Jeffrey Osborne	Don't Stop	A&M	SP-5017	Heart	Stomach	Aerobics	132
Magic Fly	Kebekelektrik	LP Single	TK Disco	NONE	Heart	Stomach	Aerobics	132
Gloria	Laura Branigan	Branigan	Atlantic	K-50772	Heart	Stomach	Aerobics	132
Beauty and the Beast	Love and Kisses	How Much I Love You	Casablanca	NBLP-7063	Heart	Stomach	Aerobics	132
How Much, How Much I Love You	Love and Kisses	How Much I Love You	Casablanca	NBLP-7063	Heart	Stomach	Aerobics	132
I've Found Love	Love and Kisses	Love and Kisses	Casablanca	NBLP-7091	Heart	Stomach	Aerobics	132

* The primary body area for which this song is good.
** The secondary body area for which this song is good.

ARTIST	ALBUM	REC. CO.	NUMBER	BODY/ONE*	BODY/TWO**	SEGMENT	BPM
So Many Men—So Little Time — Miguel Brown	LP Single	TSR	NONE	Heart	Stomach	Aerobics	132
Keep On Jumpin' — Musique	Keep On Jumpin'	Prelude	PRL-12158	Heart	Stomach	Aerobics	132
The Beach — New Order	LP Single	Factory	FACTUS1OA	Heart	Stomach	Aerobics	132
I Go to Rio — Pablo Cruise	Worlds Away	A&M	SP-4697	Heart	Stomach	Aerobics	132
Coming Out of Hiding — Pamela Stanley	LP Single	TSR	TSR-830	Heart	Stomach	Aerobics	132
Do Ya Wanna Funk — Pat Cowley & Sylvester	(Single)	Megatone	MT-102	Heart	Stomach	Aerobics	132
Jump for My Love — Pointer Sisters	Break Out	Planet	BXL1-4705	Heart	Stomach	Aerobics	132
Turn On the Action — Quincy Jones	The Dude	A&M	SP-3721	Heart	Stomach	Aerobics	132
The Hills of Katmandu — Tantra	Tantra/The Double Album	Importe-12	MP-310	Heart	Stomach	Aerobics	132
Wishbone — Tantra	Tantra/The Double Album	Importe-12	MP-310	Heart	Stomach	Aerobics	132
Disco Inferno — The Tramps	Saturday Night Fever	RSO	RS-24001	Heart	Stomach	Aerobics	132
Latin Odyssey — Voyage	Voyage	Marlin	2213	Heart	Stomach	Aerobics	132
Orient Express — Voyage	Voyage	Marlin	2213	Heart	Stomach	Aerobics	132
Could It Be Magic — Donna Summer	A Love Trilogy	Oasis	OCLP-5004	Stomach	Heart	Aerobics	132
This Is Hot — Pamela Stanley	This Is Hot	EMI	SW-17011	Stomach	Heart	Aerobics	132
It Ain't Necessarily So — Bronski Beat	The Age of Consent	MCA	MCA-5538	Legs	Back	Cool-Down	132
Heatwave — Bronski Beat	The Age of Consent	MCA	MCA-5538	Buttocks	Stomach	Tone-Up	132
Panic — Cerrone	Cerrone 6—Panic	Malligator	ULP/19	Buttocks	Stomach	Tone-Up	132
Philadelphia Freedom — Elton John	Greatest Hits #2	MCA	3027	Buttocks	Stomach	Tone-Up	132
Pinball Wizard — Elton John	Greatest Hits #2	MCA	3027	Buttocks	Stomach	Tone-Up	132
Faster Than the Speed of Light — Giorgio	From Here to Eternity	Casablanca	NBLP-7065	Buttocks	Stomach	Tone-Up	132
Crime Pays — Hall & Oates	H2O	RCA	Afl1-4383	Buttocks	Stomach	Tone-Up	132
Body — Jacksons	Victory	Epic	QE-38946	Buttocks	Stomach	Tone-Up	132
Memory (Theme from "Cats") — Menage	LP Single	Profile	PRO-70228	Buttocks	Stomach	Tone-Up	132
Come With Me — Donna Summer	A Love Trilogy	Oasis	OCLP-5004	Legs	Stomach	Tone-Up	132
Friends — Bette Midler	The Divine Miss M	Atlantic	SD-7238	Stomach	Buttocks	Tone-Up	132
Uptown Girl — Billy Joel	An Innocent Man	Columbia	QC-38837	Stomach	Buttocks	Tone-Up	132
Run to You — Bryan Adams	Reckless	A&M	SP-5013	Stomach	Buttocks	Tone-Up	132
You Know What to Do — Carly Simon	Hello Big Man	WB	23886-1	Stomach	Buttocks	Tone-Up	132
Say You'll Be Mine — Christopher Cross	Christopher Cross	WB	BSK-3383	Stomach	Buttocks	Tone-Up	132

PART THREE

CHAPTER EIGHT

AN OUNCE OF PREVENTION

He will be the slave of many masters who is his body's slave.

—Seneca (1st century)

When you exercise, you are tearing down your body tissues and using ILLNESS up energy. That's just what you want, unless you have a systemic illness, such as the flu, which will retard tissue regeneration and sap you of energy. If you come down with an illness that attacks your entire system, it is probably best to lay off your exercise program until you feel better.[1] (You should not be susceptible to many colds or cases of the flu, though, if you are working out with regular aerobic exercise and eating right.)

If you have a localized illness, such as a headache or sore throat caused by air pollution, it should not affect your workout. In fact, exercise may actually make you feel better. The same goes for menstrual cramps: Unless they are very severe, exercise will alleviate much of the discomfort.

Bad Backs

For 20 years, I lived with a constant, nagging backache, which I as- PAIN AND sumed was caused by the hours I spent bent over a camera every day, INJURIES working as a fashion photographer. I thought it was an insolvable problem, since I wasn't about to give up my livelihood just because of a little pain. Over the years, I saw doctors and chiropractors, and took medication prescribed by the doctors to ease my pain. I also probably abused alcohol in my effort to rid myself of the pain.

Not once in 20 years of suffering did anyone tell me that my stomach muscles hold up my back. I found this out when I started to do aerobics and stomach exercises. At first my back hurt worse than ever, but my stomach muscles got stronger and stronger, and now, at 51, I no longer have any back pain at all.

Arthritis

Arthritis sufferers should not shy away from exercise. As long as working out does not increase your discomfort, go right ahead and enjoy yourself.[2] You will reap the same physical, mental, and emotional benefits as anyone else. And it's possible that the endorphins released during exercise may lessen your pain.

Injuries Incurred During Exercise

When I first started doing aerobics, I used to get a minor injury a week. I thought this was normal for an out-of-shape middle-aged man. Nothing could be further from the truth.

First of all, I was working out in a club that held its aerobics class on

AN OUNCE OF PREVENTION 195

a concrete floor. In all fairness, they did have a carpet over the concrete, with the normal rug pad under the carpet. But that is certainly not enough.

My advice is to work out on a wood floor, if possible. If not, then I suggest you go to your nearest gym supply house and buy an athletic mat like the ones made for gymnastics. The one I have is made by GSC, is 1½ inches thick and is made of heavy-duty, stiff foam plastic.

I also make sure to always do aerobics in my New Balance running shoes to give my feet maximum support and my legs maximum shock absorption. I'm interested in making my workout as easy and safe as I possibly can, so that I can get up and do it again the next day. Working out at home as I do now, I am in competition with no one, so I am never tempted to push myself to the point of injury. Injuries that take even a day or two to mend would take me out of the routine I have worked so hard to establish.

At all costs, you must try not to allow yourself to lose the conditioning that you have built up. And that means that if you have shin splints that prevent you from running, you should do other exercises until you heal. Never give up exercising entirely, even for just a few days. There have been many times that my hip or leg was bothering me, so I ran on one leg or at least I distributed the weight equally on both feet. (I would do the exercises in which you land on both feet at the same time—jumping jacks, etc.—if one hip or leg was hurting.) There are times, certainly, when it hurts too much to run on your injury. Then I do any exercise that can be done fast (remember any exercise done fast enough can be aerobic) or I ride my bicycle.

Shin Splints

Shin splints are by far the most common injury for people who do aerobics and who run. Shin splints are tendons on the front of your leg that have pulled away from their protective sheath. They are caused by overexercising, from exercising when you are out of shape, from running on concrete, or from working out without the proper running shoes.

Warm up your legs with stretches before you work out; never overdo it; never run on concrete; never neglect to wear the proper shoes. But sometimes, even with the proper precautions, you will get a shin splint. If you do, here is the way to get well again.

Massage the front of your leg from your kneecap to your ankle in a sliding motion to smooth out the sheath that encloses the tendon. This can be done whenever you're sitting down, even at the office or riding to work on the train or when your car is stopped at a traffic light. Five minutes at a time, five or six times a day, should do it.

The tendon can also be moved if you rotate your foot in a circular motion when you are sitting. Or you can move your foot by pointing your toes up and down (like a ballet dancer) while you are sitting. These exercises can also be done almost anywhere during the day or even when you are lying down at night.

In addition to massage, try applying heat before you stretch, then ice down after your workout and before your cool-down stretch.

If you use these methods, you should be patched up in a couple of weeks.

(However, if you experience shin pain while exercising, plus numbness in the foot, stop and call your doctor for an appointment.)[3]

Knees

Knees, the largest joints in the body, are the most common site of pain in runners. They are vulnerable to injury and inflammation in just about any aerobic exercise.

If your knees start to hurt, apply ice after working out and go easy on them for a day or two. Keep up the ice treatment for three to five days. Significant improvement can be expected in about a week. The problem is most likely that your knees are acting as shock absorbers, because your thigh muscles aren't strong enough. An orthopedic doctor can show you how to remedy this by building thigh strength with weight training.

You'll know if your knees are really injured if the pain is consistent and swelling appears, if pain persists long after you finish working out, if your knees buckle under you, if you hear any noises emanating from the knee as you move it, or if the pain just plain gets worse.[4]

If possible, seek treatment at a sports medicine clinic for any orthopedic problem. The doctors at such centers are committed to returning you to your workout program, not sending you to the couch to watch TV. They make an effort to keep up with all the latest research, and, most importantly, actually practice what they preach. These doctors are athletic themselves, and that's the reason most of them decided to specialize in sports medicine.

Bursitis

Bursitis is a common complaint for active people. Technically an inflammation of the bursa (a small, fluid-filled sac that cushions your tendons from rubbing against your bones), bursitis can be caused by overuse or misalignment. Trouble spots are shoulders, hips, and knees.

The best thing to do if you feel a burning sensation is to apply ice after you exercise. As with knee problems, if the symptoms don't show improvement after five days of ice treatment and coddling the inflamed part of the body, call your doctor.[5]

Ice and Heat

The two standard remedies for injury are applying ice or heat to the site; the critical thing is to make sure you apply the *right* one, at the right time. If you misdiagnose your problem, or forget which goes with which type of injury, you will exacerbate your problem instead of relieving it.

Try to remember this: Ice is for burning; heat is for stiffness. (If you aren't sure which one you've got, and are in real pain, call a doctor before you do yourself any damage.)

Ice combats inflammation (which really seems like a small fire burning under the skin; in fact, you can feel the heat coming off the inflamed spot with your hand), and it should be applied *after* you exercise. Your joints, tendons, and muscles can all suffer from inflammation.

I recommend buying liquid "cold packs" at your sporting-goods or drug store to keep in your freezer, in case you overwork yourself and suffer inflammation. They freeze nearly to ice, yet stay flexible enough to wrap around a knee or elbow. They can also be secured inside an elastic bandage so they stay in place. (Ace makes a very good cold pack.)

Ice should be applied as soon as you feel the burn and should be left on for about 10 minutes. Make sure that the ice does not come into direct contact with your skin (put a thin cloth under the ice if you are not wearing leotards or sweat pants) or you will blister from the extreme cold.

You will be able to feel the heat of the inflammation die down as the ice does its job.

If you are at your health club and can't get hold of a cup of ice from a vending machine, take a shower and turn the coldest possible water right on the burn. It isn't as good as ice, but it will help till you get home.

Heat is for warming up tight muscles and tendons. It is really a preventive treatment and should be applied *before* your workout. You can use a commercial heat rub like Ben-Gay, a heating pad, or a hot tub.

Heat expands the molecules in your cells, eases muscle cramps, relieves stiffness, and gets your body limbered up and ready to exercise.[6]

Aspirin

Aspirin is a wonderful painkiller if you really need one. Aspirin reduces inflammation, thereby cutting down on the pain at its source and healing overworked muscles or joints. Most people do not know, however, that aspirin is absorbed into the bloodstream through the intestines, so that the pain-killing effect does not start for about an hour. Consequently, you should not wait until you are hurting really badly to take an aspirin or two—by the same token, don't be impatient and start popping three or four when relief isn't instantaneous.

If you are suffering from inflammation, take two aspirin an hour before you work out. That way it is in your system, reducing the inflammation, as you start to exercise.

I recommend Ecotrin, a coated aspirin that passes through the stomach before dissolving in the intestine. This safeguards against irritation of the stomach lining. Tylenol, and other aspirin substitutes, will not reduce inflammation. I also recommend buying the low-dose Ecotrin, as that allows you to control your dosage easily.

Chances are that if you follow my exercise plan, you will never need a stronger painkiller than aspirin, and that infrequently. Our Aerobicise program was designed to expose you to the least possibility of injury for the maximum return in fitness of any exercise program.

WHAT TO WEAR

You don't need to rush right out and invest in designer leotards, tights, leg warmers, elastic belts, headbands, wristbands, etc., in order to be appropriately dressed for the Aerobicise workouts. All you need is loose, comfortable clothing that will allow you maximum movement. Leotards are great, but you can also wear shorts and T shirts if you like. (A well-fitted leotard will offer enough breast support for the small- to average-sized woman; bras should be worn under shirts.) As far as your body goes, the object is to be comfortable.

Your mind is another matter. Sometimes we need to use whatever psychological gimmicks we can find to spur us onward. Pretty, sexy exercise clothes can provide just the impetus you need to get past your inertia and into a workout. If knowing that you have a new outfit to put on makes you look forward to your workout, by all means go out and buy one. Whatever makes the prospect of getting in shape more appealing is a worthwhile device.

Once you are into your fitness routine, however, you'll probably feel so good about exercising that you won't need to get yourself "psyched up" to each workout with payoffs of new pink-and-lavender-striped leotards. You'll enjoy the movement and feeling of well-being so much that what you wear will seem incidental.

There are some clothing tips you may want to keep in mind, though, when starting an Aerobicise wardrobe:

Make sure the material of your clothes is appropriate to the climate of your workout room. If your room is warm, cotton is the best fabric, because it soaks up moisture and breathes well. You are better off with nylon or Lycra in a cool or air-conditioned room, for those fabrics allow perspiration to dry quickly and they keep moisture away from your skin.

Don't confuse fashion with fitness. The current vogue for leg warmers, for example, has far overreached what was originally a fairly specific practical application. Now ubiquitous on the streets of every city in America, leg warmers were manufactured for dancers, who wore them to keep their legs warm (their *legs*, not their ankles) and ward off stiffness, increasing flexibility in cold rooms before their circulation got going and did the job itself.

You can certainly use them the way dancers do, for keeping the legs warm at the beginning of your workout.

As far as other accessories go, none of them are necessary, but you may find some of them appealing. Sweatbands can keep perspiration out of your eyes and your hair off of your face, for instance; and elastic belts can be a helpful visual aid for proper hip placement. Make sure you don't wear either too tight, however.

Whether you opt for leotards, with or without tights, or shorts and a shirt, there is one part of your workout outfit for which there is no substitute: socks. You *must* be sure to wear socks with your shoes. (I recommend cotton, as it breathes the best.) Bare feet or feet covered only by thin nylon will slip around, unbalance you, and probably blister.

There is one other ironclad rule: Don't expose yourself to the risk of a chill by peeling off layers of clothing while you work out and then neglecting to put them back on again when you finish exercising.

If you are working out in a cool room, it's a very good idea to wear a sweatshirt, or anything else you have that's both warm and nonrestricting, when you begin to exercise. As your circulation goes into high gear and you begin to perspire, you'll want to strip down to your leotard or T shirt. That's fine, because your body will be nice and warm by then. But when you go into the cool-down phase of your workout, your circulation will slow and your body will do just what that part of the routine is named for—cool down. That's when you should put that sweatshirt back on, particularly if you are working out in an air-conditioned or drafty room.

Shoes should be chosen for protection against injury, not for fashion. **SHOES** I recommend New Balance running shoes for maximum cushioning effect and little weight. There are many other running shoes, of course, that will do the trick. New Balance just happens to be my personal favorite.

CHAPTER NINE

THE FOUNTAIN OF YOUTH

For when I was a babe and wept and slept, Time crept, When I was a boy and laughed and talked, Time walked; Then when the years saw me a man, Time ran, But as I older grew, Time flew.
    —Guy Pentreath

The reason for this apparent speeding up of time is that our organic processes tend to slow down as we grow older, so that compared with them, civil time, as registered by the clock and the calendar, appears to go even faster.

    —G. J. Whitrow, The Natural
    Philosophy of Time

The older you get, the faster time seems to go. When you are old, the **SLOWING** days speed by as if in an hour. What a shame that is. Aerobic exercise **DOWN** is the only way to speed up your metabolism so that you feel younger **FATHER** and the days are longer to enjoy. That is one of the best reasons I can **TIME** think of for doing aerobic exercise. And it just might be that the diseases of the aged are triggered by the slowing down of one's metabolism.

The largest single cause of cancer in the world is smoking. The link **SMOKING** between smoking and cancer is overwhelming. Thinking you won't get cancer from smoking is the most fanciful thinking you can do.

One of the reasons smoking causes cancer is the amount of radiation we get from tobacco smoke. Another reason is that carbon monoxide (the poisonous product of burning) is carried into our blood, where it displaces the oxygen that is necessary for our very existence.

This year, each person in the United States will receive an average of about 80 millirems of radiation from natural sources and about 100 millirems from man-made sources. Medical technicians accumulate about three times the dose of the average person, or approximately 540 millirems of radiation per year. A smoker of one and a half packs of cigarettes per day receives *8,000 millirems per year!*[1]

Stop committing suicide. Stop smoking now!

Bruce Ames, chairman of the biochemistry department at the Univer- **DIET AND** sity of California, Berkeley, is one of the world's leading cancer re- **CANCER** searchers. (He developed the test that is used for detecting mutagens [cancer-causing substances] more than a decade ago.) Ames has recently switched the emphasis of his attack on cancer from man-made chemicals to the toxins that are present in everyday foods.

Ames has determined that man-made chemicals "actually are a drop in the bucket compared with the number of natural carcinogens in the environment." He is now convinced that the "bulk of cancer isn't coming from man-made chemicals. All the evidence suggests that it's coming from other sources." Where do these natural toxins come from? Nature makes them to protect itself; it puts toxic substances in plants to fend off predators—bacteria, fungus, insects, and animals. Don't despair. We'd all have been dead a long time ago if nature, in its infinite balance, didn't have just as many anticarcinogens up its sleeve as carcinogens. These anticarcinogens, also known as antioxidants, are Vitamin A, Vitamin C, Vitamin E, and selenium.[2]

The chances are you do not, and probably cannot, get enough A, C, E, and selenium from your food to fight the toxins. So, the obvious answer is to get them from vitamin supplements. It is important that you take approximately the same amount each day; the only way I know how to do that is to take premeasured doses, from a bottle.

I read *Selenium as Food and Medicine*, by Dr. Richard A. Passwater. This book made selenium (which is a fundamental element) sound like the wonder drug of the '80s in its ability to prevent cancer, heart disease, arthritis, radiation, cystic fibrosis, muscular dystrophy, and sexual dysfunction.[3]

I was a disbeliever, even though the evidence presented was from the most credible sources available as of 1980, the year of its publication. Then I remembered a line from Bruce Ames's research: "Thus, Vitamin E, which was discovered 60 years ago as a fertility factor, and other antioxidants such as selenium, may help to engender and to protect the next generation."[4]

With my newfound respect for selenium, I immediately did a search with my computer, and found 1,699 references on selenium since 1981. Obviously, lots of researchers were spending lots of money on learning about selenium, and the research showed that selenium, usually in combination with Vitamin E, could prevent cancer. Selenium may be one of the most important nutrients you can take to prevent disease and to keep you healthy longer. I personally take 100 mcg of it, in the form of selenium from yeast, every day. (See Nutrient Chart, page 210.)

SKIN CANCER   Skin cancer is also prevalent in our society, and can be guarded against by avoiding prolonged exposure to the sun. Research shows that truck drivers get cancer on their left arm, which is exposed to the sun as they drive along with that arm hanging out the window. Studies show a high percentage of those working out of doors contract skin cancer.[5]

The use of tanning booths has become so widespread that the incidence of skin cancer is probably on the increase. The skin-cancer-inducing radiation received in getting a tan inside a tanning booth may be as much as *twice* that of tanning in natural sunlight.[6]

You should certainly not avoid sunlight, because it is very important to your body. Several studies done in Sweden show that the Swedes do not metabolize calcium as well as Americans. The evidence points to sunlight as the reason for this. Sweden is so far north that the light is shifted toward the red end of the spectrum, much as a sunset is, because

maintenance of a healthy nervous system. Deficiency of vitamin B_{12} results in pernicious anemia.

MULTIMINERAL: My brand is called Super Multi-Minerals. Although my multivitamin contains many of the same minerals, this supplement gives me much larger amounts of them.

The minerals and their doses are: 500 mg calcium; 250 mg magnesium; 75 mcg iodine; 15 mg iron; 11.25 mg zinc; 0.5 mg copper; 5 mg manganese; 47 mg potassium; 50 mg betaine; 200 IU vitamin D3; 2.5 mcg selenium; 0.05 mg chromium.

Minerals are essential for the proper composition of body fluids, for bone and blood formation, and for healthy nerve function. Women of childbearing age must be especially careful to get enough iron, or anemia may result. My formula should be sufficient for the average woman, but if chronic weakness and fatigue are experienced, a blood test to detect anemia, and an increase in iron supplements, could be in order.

VITAMIN C POWDER: Because I really believe in the power of vitamin C, I take it three ways every day: as part of my multivitamin, in this powdered supplement, and in a C-complex tablet. I use the Great Earth brand, which is a fine, crystalline vitamin C powder, one-quarter teaspoon of which equals 1250 mg. You just mix it in a glass of juice or any beverage and drink it a couple of times a day. Powdered C is preferable for anyone sensitive to acid, because it is already dissolved when it goes down and is therefore less likely to irritate the stomach.

SUPER C COMPLEX: My C complex is a timed-release, 1000 mg pill in a base of natural rose hips. On days when it's inconvenient to mix up and drink my powdered C, I know I'm getting the basic dose I need with this supplement.

VITAMIN E, PLUS ANTIOXIDANTS: Called Oxy.E.400, this supplement contains 400 IU of vitamin E; 100 mg of C; 1000 IU of A; 100 IU of D_3; and the following minerals: calcium, magnesium, potassium, zinc, manganese, lecithin, selenium, and chromium.

The vitamins and minerals in this tablet combine to be superb antioxidants, excellent for combating the toxins that cause cancer and other diseases.

VITAMIN A (BETA CAROTENE): This gives you the equivalent of 25,000 IU of vitamin A, 250 mg of vitamin C, 60 IU of vitamin E, and 60 mcg of selenium in a high-potency, concentrated base of beta carotene-rich vegetables: carrots, tomatoes, beets, spinach, lettuce, red and green peppers, cabbage, cauliflower, Brussels sprouts, alfalfa, and parsley. Beta carotene is converted to vitamin A once inside the system.

SELENIUM: I believe selenium is the "wonder mineral." It guards against cancer, heart disease, arthritis, the effects of radiation, cystic fibrosis, muscular dystrophy, and sexual dysfunction. Selenium may be one of the most important nutrients you can take to prevent disease and to keep you healthy longer.[16]

CHOLINE AND INOSITOL COMPOUND: Choline transforms into acetylcholine, the chemical neurotransmitter that telegraphs messages from one brain cell to another. Without these neurotransmitters you would be unable to learn, remember, sleep, move, or emote. You would cease to function.

An experiment at M.I.T. showed that students taking 3 grams of choline a day experienced improved memory and learning ability; their brains were literally transmitting messages and information faster and better.

Choline is also vital to proper kidney and liver function. In combination with inositol, it forms lecithin, which metabolizes fat and cholesterol.

Inositol is a sugar required for muscle cell growth. It may be useful in arthritis treatment and hair-loss reduction.

The compound I take contains 250 mg each of choline and inositol.

NUTRIENT FORMULA: VITAMINS AND MINERALS

The following recommendations are for adults, over 20 years of age.

Multivitamin with vitamin A	10,000 IU
Multimineral with calcium	500 MG
Vitamin C, timed release	1,000 MG
Vitamin C, powdered in fruit juice	1,000 MG
Vitamin E (dry type)	800 IU
Choline and inositol, each	1,000 MG
Beta carotene, equivalent of vitamin A activity	25,000 IU
Selenium from yeast	100 MCG

This experimental formula is not recommended for children or pregnant women, nor is it meant as a substitute for prescription drugs. If you are under medical treatment, make sure you consult with your doctor before beginning a vitamin and nutrient supplement plan. We have made no attempt to evaluate the safety of this formula. It is my personal formula, the one that works for me. I recommend you go to a reputable health food store and talk to one of their experts on vitamins and nutrition. They should be able to help you design your own formula for nutrition.

There is a great deal you can do to preserve your youth. The choice is yours: You can start living today. The first thing to do when you get up tomorrow is exercise, and start caring for the only body you will ever have. The strenuous exercise described in *Aerobicise* is the central step toward being part of the new, healthy generation. It is probably the single greatest thing you can do to improve your life.

APPENDIX

Fat and Fiber Charts

The following charts show you the fat and fiber content of common foods, broken down into nine categories: dairy; fats and oils; fish, meat, and poultry; fruit and fruit products; grain products; legumes, nuts, and seeds; sugars and sweets; vegetables and vegetable products; and miscellaneous items, including fast foods. The foods are listed in average portion sizes for easy reference. Liquids are given in fluid oz. and solids by weight.

The basic formula is this: Eat as little fat as you can. Choose foods as high in fiber as possible.

We recommend that you try to keep your fat intake under 20 grams per day and your fiber intake as much over 15 grams as you can.

FAT CONTENT

FOOD	PORTION	GRAMS OF FAT
Eggnog	1 cup	19.00
Ricotta cheese—whole milk	½ cup	16.00
Ice cream—Rich (16% fat)	½ cup	12.00
Ice cream—soft (frozen custard)	½ cup	11.50
Cream cheese	1 oz	10.00
Ricotta cheese—skim milk	½ cup	9.50
Vanilla milk shake	11 oz	9.00
Chocolate malted milk	1 cup	9.00
Camembert cheese	1.3 oz	9.00
Cheddar cheese	1 oz	9.00
Parmesan cheese (grated)	1 oz	9.00
Processed American cheese	1 oz	9.00
Chocolate milk shake	10.6 oz	8.00
Chocolate milk	1 cup	8.00
Blue cheese	1 oz	8.00
Provolone cheese	1 oz	8.00
Romano cheese	1 oz	8.00
Swiss cheese	1 oz	8.00
Whole milk—3.3% fat	1 cup	8.00
Baked custard	½ cup	7.50
Mozzarella cheese—whole milk	1 oz	7.00
Processed Swiss cheese	1 oz	7.00
Processed cheese food	1 oz	7.00
Ice cream—regular (11% fat)	½ cup	7.00
Yogurt—whole milk	8 oz	7.00
Egg, scrambled with milk and butter	1 egg	7.00
Chocolate pudding	½ cup	6.00
Processed cheese spread	1 oz	6.00
Cream, heavy whipping	1 tbsp	6.00
Eggs, whole large	1 egg	6.00
Egg, large poached	1 egg	6.00
Cottage cheese (4% fat)	½ cup	5.00
Milk—2% fat	1 cup	5.00
Vanilla pudding	½ cup	5.00
Plain yogurt (lowfat milk)	8 oz	4.00
Fruit yogurt (lowfat)	8 oz	3.00
Light cream (for coffee)	1 tbsp	3.00
Sour cream	1 tbsp	3.00
Ice milk—4.3% fat	½ cup	3.00
Cottage cheese (lowfat—2%)	½ cup	2.00
Half-and-half	1 tbsp	2.00
Buttermilk	1 cup	2.00
Sherbet—2% fat	½ cup	2.00
Whipped cream topping	1 tbsp	1.00
Imitation cream, powdered	1 tsp	1.00
Imitation cream—pressure top	1 tbsp	1.00

DAIRY PRODUCTS, LISTED BY FAT CONTENT

FATS AND OILS, LISTED BY FAT CONTENT	FOOD	PORTION	GRAMS OF FAT
	Salad dressing—Italian	2 tbsp	18.00
	Salad dressing—Thousand Island	2 tbsp	16.00
	Salad Dressing—blue cheese	2 tbsp	16.00
	Corn oil	1 tbsp	14.00
	Olive oil	1 tbsp	14.00
	Peanut oil	1 tbsp	14.00
	Safflower/Soybean oil	1 tbsp	14.00
	Cooking fats—vegetable	1 tbsp	13.00
	Lard	1 tbsp	13.00
	Salad dressing—French	2 tbsp	12.00
	Butter	1 tbsp	12.00
	Margarine	1 tbsp	12.00
	Salad dressing—mayonnaise	1 tbsp	11.00
	Butter, whipped	1 tbsp	8.00
	Salad dressing—tartar	1 tbsp	8.00
	Butter	1 pat	4.00
	Margarine	1 pat	4.00
	Butter, whipped	1 pat	3.00
	Salad dressing—low cal.	2 tbsp	2.00

FISH, MEAT, AND POULTRY, LISTED BY FAT CONTENT	FOOD	PORTION	GRAMS OF FAT
	Beef, roast, rib—lean & fat	3 oz	33.00
	Lamb chop/rib, broiled—lean & fat	3.1 oz	32.00
	Canned ham—luncheon	2 slices	30.00
	Beef, sirloin steak, broiled—lean & fat	3 oz	27.00
	Pork chop/loin, broiled—lean & fat	2.7 oz	25.00
	Pork roast—lean & fat	3 oz	24.00
	Chicken potpie—frozen	1 pie	23.25
	Lamb, shoulder, roasted—lean & fat	3 oz	23.00
	Beef potpie—frozen	1 pie	22.50
	Ham, roasted—lean & fat	3 oz	19.00
	Chop suey with beef & pork	1 cup	17.00
	Chicken a la king	½ cup	17.00
	Ground beef, broiled—21% fat	3 oz	17.00
	Chili con carne—canned	1 cup	16.00
	Beef, simmered or roasted—lean & fat	3 oz	16.00
	Lamb, leg, roasted—lean & fat	3 oz	16.00
	Bologna	2 slices	16.00
	Braunschweiger	2 slices	16.00
	Frankfurter	1 frank	15.00
	Veal, rib, roasted—no bone	3 oz	14.00
	Corned beef hash—canned	½ cup	12.50
	Brown & serve sausages	2 links	12.00
	Pork link sausage	2 links	12.00
	Salami—dry type	1 oz	12.00
	Beef & vegetable stew	1 cup	11.00
	Ocean perch, breaded, fried	1 fillet	11.00
	Tuna salad	½ cup	11.00
	Ground beef, broiled—10% fat	3 oz	10.00
	Corned beef—canned	3 oz	10.00
	Boiled ham—luncheon	2 slices	10.00
	Pork roast—lean	2.4 oz	10.00
	Sardines—canned in oil	3 oz	9.00
	Shrimp—French fried	3 oz	9.00
	Lamb chop/rib, broiled—lean	3 oz	9.00
	Beef liver, fried	3 oz	9.00

Food	Portion	Grams of Fat
Pork chop/loin, broiled—lean	2 oz	9.00
Veal cutlet	3 oz	9.00
Chicken & noodles	½ cup	9.00
Scallops, breaded, fried	6 scallops	8.00
Bacon, broiled or fried—crisp	2 strips	8.00
Beef, roast, rib—lean	3 oz	7.80
Tuna, canned, oil drained	3 oz	7.00
Salami—cooked type	1 oz	7.00
Chicken, broiled	6.2 oz (½ broiler)	7.00
Turkey, dark meat—no skin	4 pieces	7.00
Beef, sirloin steak, broiled—lean	3 oz	6.00
Lamb, shoulder, roasted—lean	2.3 oz	6.00
Vienna sausages	2 sausages	6.00
Turkey, light meat—no skin	4 pieces	6.00
Haddock, breaded, fried	3 oz	5.00
Salmon, pink—canned	3 oz	5.00
Beef, simmered or roasted—lean	2.5 oz	5.00
Beef heart, braised—lean	3 oz	5.00
Lamb, leg, roasted—lean	2.5 oz	5.00
Chicken chow mein	½ cup	5.00
Bluefish, baked with butter	3 oz	4.00
Deviled ham—canned	1 tbsp	4.00
Chicken, drumstick, fried	1.3 oz	4.00
Fish sticks, breaded	1-oz stick	3.00
Oysters, raw, meat only	½ cup	2.00
King crab meat—canned	½ cup	1.50
Clams, raw, meat only	3 oz	1.00
Clams—canned	3 oz	1.00
Shrimp—canned meat	3 oz	1.00

FRUITS AND FRUIT PRODUCTS, LISTED BY FAT CONTENT

FOOD	PORTION	GRAMS OF FAT
Avocado (California)	½ avocado	18.50
Avocado (Florida)	½ avocado	16.50
Pear, with skin	1 pear	1.00
Apples, raw	1 apple	1.00
Watermelon, raw	1 wedge	1.00
Blackberries	½ cup	0.50
Apricots, dried, uncooked	½ cup	0.50
Blueberries, raw	½ cup	0.50
Pears—canned in heavy syrup	½ cup	0.50
Raspberries, sweet—frozen	5 oz.	0.50
Raspberries, raw	½ cup	0.50
Prunes, dried, cooked	½ cup	0.50
Strawberries, sweet—frozen	5 oz	0.50
Strawberries, raw	½ cup	0.50
Cranberry sauce, sweet—canned	¼ cup	0.25
Strawberries—frozen	½ cup	0.25

GRAIN PRODUCTS, LISTED BY FAT CONTENT

FOOD	PORTION	GRAMS OF FAT
Pecan pie	1 piece	27.00
Macaroni & cheese	1 cup	22.00
Mince pie	1 piece	16.00
Blueberry pie	1 piece	15.00
Pumpkin pie	1 piece	15.00
Apple pie	1 piece	15.00
Cherry pie	1 piece	15.00

Danish pastry, plain	1 pastry	15.00
Peach pie	1 piece	14.00
Custard pie	1 piece	14.00
Banana cream pie	1 piece	12.00
Sheet cake, no icing	1 piece	12.00
Spaghetti, with tomato sauce and meat	1 cup	12.00
Lemon meringue pie	1 piece	12.00
Doughnut, glazed	1 doughnut	11.00
Roll, hard	1 roll	10.00
Pound cake	1 piece	10.00
Macaroons	2 cookies	9.00
Chocolate chip cookies	4 cookies	9.00
Cookies, sandwich type	4 cookies	9.00
Devil's food cake, with icing	1 piece	8.00
Cake, white, with icing	1 piece	8.00
Cake, yellow, with icing	1 piece	8.00
Oatmeal cookies	4 cookies	8.00
Waffles, from mix with eggs & milk	1 waffle	8.00
Coffee cake	1 piece	7.00
Vanilla wafer cookies	10 cookies	6.00
Toaster pastries	1 pastry	6.00
Boston cream cake	1 piece	6.00
Brownies	1 brownie	6.00
Cupcake, with chocolate icing	1 cupcake	5.00
Biscuit, homemade	1 biscuit	5.00
Doughnut, plain	1 doughnut	5.00
Bran muffin, homemade	1 muffin	4.00
Pizza, small, with cheese	1 piece	4.00
Blueberry muffin	1 muffin	4.00
Corn muffin	1 muffin	4.00
Muffin, plain	1 muffin	4.00
Roll, submarine	1 roll	4.00
Gingerbread cake	1 piece	4.00
Sponge cake	1 piece	4.00
Fig-bar cookie	4 cookies	3.00
Pretzel, twisted	10 pretzels	3.00
Clover roll	1 roll	3.00
Cupcake, no icing	1 cupcake	3.00
Oatmeal	1 cup	2.00
Bagel, egg	1 bagel	2.00
Egg noodles—cooked	1 cup	2.00
Popcorn, with oil & salt	1 cup	2.00
Pancakes, buckwheat	1 pancake	2.00
Roll, hamburger	1 roll	2.00
Roll, brown & serve	1 roll	2.00
Gingersnap cookies	4 cookies	2.00
Pancakes, plain	1 pancake	2.00
Fruitcake, dark with raisins	1 slice	2.00
Cereal, bran, with raisins	1 cup	1.00
Cereal, bran flakes 40%	1 cup	1.00
Cereal, shredded wheat	½ cup	1.00
Cereal, puffed oats	1 cup	1.00
Bread, wheat, soft—toasted	1 slice	1.00
Bread, raisin	1 slice	1.00
Bagel, water	1 bagel	1.00
Graham crackers	2 crackers	1.00
Macaroni noodles, cooked	1 cup	1.00
Saltine crackers	4 crackers	1.00
Spaghetti noodles, cooked	1 cup	1.00
Bread, wheat, firm—18 slices/loaf	1 slice	1.00
Bread, wheat, soft—16 slices/loaf	1 slice	1.00

Bread, white, firm—34 slices/loaf	1 slice	1.00
Bread, white, soft—24 slices/loaf	1 slice	1.00
Bread, white, soft—18 slices/loaf	1 slice	1.00
Cereal, wheat	1 cup	1.00
Cereal, puffed corn	1 cup	1.00
Cereal, wheat germ	¼ cup	0.50

FOOD	PORTION	GRAMS OF FAT
Pecans, chopped	¼ cup	21.00
Walnuts, English	¼ cup	19.25
Peanuts, salted, roasted in oil	¼ cup	18.00
Filberts	¼ cup	18.00
Almonds, chopped	¼ cup	17.50
Sunflower seeds	¼ cup	17.25
Almonds, slivered	¼ cup	17.25
Pumpkin or Squash seeds	¼ cup	16.25
Cashew nuts, roasted in oil	¼ cup	16.00
Brazil nuts, shelled	1 oz	9.50
Beans, with franks—canned	½ cup	9.00
Peanut butter	1 tbsp	8.00
Coconut, shredded	¼ cup	7.00
Beans, with pork/sweet sauce—canned	½ cup	4.00
Beans, with pork & tomato sauce—canned	½ cup	3.50
Black-eyed peas	½ cup	0.50
Lima beans	½ cup	0.50
Beans, navy, dry-cooked	½ cup	0.50
Peas, split, dry—cooked	½ cup	0.50
Beans, red kidney—canned	½ cup	0.50

LEGUMES, NUTS, AND SEEDS, LISTED BY FAT CONTENT

FOOD	PORTION	GRAMS OF FAT
Chocolate, semisweet bits	¼ cup	15.25
Chocolate-coated peanuts	1 oz	12.00
Chocolate, plain	1 oz	9.00
Chocolate-flavored fudge syrup	1 fl oz	5.00
Caramels, plain or chocolate	1 oz	3.00
Fudge	1 oz	3.00
Chocolate-flavored syrup, thin	1 oz	1.00

SUGARS AND SWEETS, LISTED BY FAT CONTENT

FOOD	PORTION	GRAMS OF FAT
Potatoes, hash brown—frozen	½ cup	9.00
Potato chips	10 chips	8.00
French fries—cooked from raw	10 strips	7.00
Potatoes, mashed (with milk and butter)	½ cup	4.50
Potato salad	½ cup	3.50
Potatoes, mashed—from dehydrated	½ cup	3.50
Sweet potato, candied	1 piece	3.00
Tomato catsup	1 oz	1.00
Corn, sweet, cream-style—canned	½ cup	1.00
Corn, sweet, wet—canned	½ cup	1.00
Sweet potato, boiled, peeled	1 potato	1.00
Corn, sweet—cooked from raw	1 ear	1.00
Bean sprouts—cooked	1 cup	0.90
Broccoli—cooked	1 stalk	0.50
Brussels sprouts, cooked from raw	1 cup	0.50
Broccoli, frozen—cooked	1 cup	0.50
Peas, green—canned	½ cup	0.50
Pumpkin—canned	½ cup	0.50
Parsnips—cooked	½ cup	0.50

VEGETABLES AND VEGETABLE PRODUCTS, LISTED BY FAT CONTENT

Sweet potato—canned	½ cup	0.50
Vegetables, mixed, frozen—cooked	½ cup	0.50
Collards—cooked	½ cup	0.50
Spinach—canned	½ cup	0.50
Corn, sweet—canned	½ cup	0.50
Spinach, chopped, frozen—cooked	½ cup	0.50
Corn, sweet, frozen—cooked	1 ear	0.50
Spinach, leaf, frozen—cooked	½ cup	0.50
Mustard greens—cooked	½ cup	0.50
Spinach—cooked from raw	½ cup	0.50
Corn, sweet, frozen—cooked	½ cup	0.50
Black-eyed peas, frozen—cooked	½ cup	0.50
Lettuce, iceberg	¼ head	0.25

MISCELLANEOUS AND FAST-FOOD ITEMS, LISTED BY FAT CONTENT

FOOD	PORTION	GRAMS OF FAT
Triple hamburger—Wendy's	1 sandwich	51.00
Double hamburger—Wendy's	1 sandwich	40.00
Big Mac—McDonald's	1 sandwich	33.00
Quarter Pounder with cheese—McDonald's	1 sandwich	31.00
Club sandwich—Arby's	1 sandwich	30.00
Single hamburger—Wendy's	1 sandwich	26.00
Fish sandwich—McDonald's	1 sandwich	25.00
Turkey deluxe—Arby's	1 sandwich	24.00
Quarter Pounder—McDonald's	1 sandwich	22.00
Burrito supreme—Taco Bell	1 burrito	22.00
Beef/cheese sandwich—Arby's	1 sandwich	22.00
Beef burrito—Taco Bell	1 burrito	21.00
Ham/cheese sandwich—Arby's	1 sandwich	17.00
Egg McMuffin—McDonald's	1 sandwich	15.00
Beef tostado—Taco Bell	1 tostado	15.00
Roast beef sandwich—Arby's	1 sandwich	15.00
Cream of mushroom soup (canned), with milk	1 cup	14.00
Cheeseburger—McDonald's	1 sandwich	14.00
Bean burrito—Taco Bell	1 burrito	12.00
Cream of mushroom soup (canned) with water	1 cup	10.00
Cream of chicken soup (canned), with milk	1 cup	10.00
Hamburger—McDonald's	1 sandwich	10.00
Taco—Taco Bell	1 taco	8.00
Cream of tomato soup (canned), with milk	1 cup	7.00
Pork/bean soup (canned), with water	1 cup	6.00
Cream of chicken soup (canned), with water	1 cup	6.00
Regular tostado—Taco Bell	1 tostado	6.00
Onion soup mix, unprepared	1½ oz	5.00
Minestrone soup (canned), with water	1 cup	3.00
Split pea soup (canned), with water	1 cup	3.00
Clam chowder, Manhattan-style (canned), with water	1 cup	3.00
Tomato soup (canned), with water	1 cup	3.00
Beef noodle soup, with water	1 cup	3.00
Barbecue sauce	1 oz	2.13
Vegetarian soup (canned), with water	1 cup	2.00
Vegetable/beef soup, with water	1 cup	2.00
Olives, green, canned, with brine	3–4 olives	2.00
Olives, black, canned	2–3 olives	2.00
Tomato vegetable soup, from mix	1 cup	1.00
Onion soup, from mix	1 cup	1.00
Chicken noodle soup, from mix	1 cup	1.00

Fiber Content

FOOD	PORTION	GRAMS OF FIBER	
Milk chocolate shake	10.6 oz	0.75	**DAIRY**
Yogurt, fruit (lowfat)	8 oz	0.27	**PRODUCTS,**
Vanilla milk shake	11 oz	0.19	**LISTED BY**
Chocolate milk	1 cup	0.15	**FIBER**
Chocolate pudding	½ cup	0.13	**CONTENT**
Chocolate malted milk	1 cup	0.08	

FOOD	PORTION	GRAMS OF FIBER	
Salad dressing—Thousand Island	2 tbsp	0.64	**FATS AND OILS,**
Salad dressing—French	2 tbsp	0.26	**LISTED BY**
Salad dressing—Italian	2 tbsp	0.06	**FIBER CONTENT**
Salad dressing—blue cheese	2 tbsp	0.03	

FOOD	PORTION	GRAMS OF FIBER	
Chili con carne—canned	1 cup	1.53	**FISH, MEAT,**
Chop suey with beef & pork	1 cup	1.25	**AND POULTRY,**
Beef & vegetable stew	1 cup	0.74	**LISTED BY**
Beef potpie—frozen	1 pie	0.63	**FIBER CONTENT**
Chicken potpie—frozen	1 pie	0.63	

FOOD	PORTION	GRAMS OF FIBER	
Avocado (Florida)	½ avocado	3.21	**FRUITS AND**
Raspberries, sweet—frozen	5 oz	3.15	**FRUIT**
Blackberries	½ cup	2.95	**PRODUCTS,**
Watermelon, raw	1 wedge	2.80	**LISTED BY**
Pear, with skin	1 pear	2.35	**FIBER**
Avocado (California)	½ avocado	2.28	**CONTENT**
Apricots, dried, uncooked	½ cup	1.92	
Raspberries, raw	½ cup	1.85	
Cantaloupe	½ melon	1.72	
Honeydew melon	1/10 melon	1.36	
Fruit cocktail—canned	1 cup	1.15	
Prunes, dried, cooked	½ cup	1.15	
Peaches, sliced, raw	1 cup	1.09	
Papayas, raw	1 cup	1.08	
Apples, raw	1 apple	1.06	
Prunes, dried, uncooked	4–5 large	1.00	
Pineapple, canned, in syrup	2 slices	1.00	
Blueberries, raw	½ cup	0.95	
Raisins, seedless	½ cup	0.95	
Strawberries, sweet—frozen	5 oz	0.90	
Dates, whole	5 dates	0.88	
Pineapple, raw	1 cup	0.84	
Orange sections, raw	1 cup	0.77	
Pears, canned in heavy syrup	½ cup	0.75	
Strawberries—frozen	½ cup	0.68	
Applesauce, unsweetened—canned	½ cup	0.65	
Apricots, raw	3 apricots	0.64	
Peaches, raw	1 peach	0.64	
Banana	1 banana	0.60	
Applesauce, sweetened—canned	½ cup	0.59	
Orange, raw	1 orange	0.56	
Pineapple, canned, in syrup	½ cup	0.55	
Cherries, raw	20 cherries	0.54	

Grapes, raw (Tokay)	20 grapes	0.54
Apricots, canned in heavy syrup	½ cup	0.52
Apple juice	1 cup	0.52
Peaches, sweetened—frozen	½ cup	0.50
Grapefruit, raw	½ grapefruit	0.48
Apricot nectar—canned	1 cup	0.48
Strawberries, raw	½ cup	0.40
Plums, raw	1 plum	0.40
Peaches, canned, in syrup	½ cup	0.37
Tangerine, raw	1 tangerine	0.30
Pineapple juice, unsweetened—canned	1 cup	0.30
Orange juice—raw or canned	1 cup	0.25
Cranberry sauce, sweetened—canned	¼ cup	0.21
Raisins, seedless	½ oz	0.20
Plums, raw	1 plum	0.20
Orange juice, from frozen	1 cup	0.13

GRAIN PRODUCTS, LISTED BY FIBER CONTENT

FOOD	PORTION	GRAMS OF FIBER
Cereal, bran, with raisins	1 cup	5.30
Cereal, bran flakes 40%	1 cup	4.80
Cereal, shredded wheat	½ cup	2.30
Cereal, oatmeal	1 cup	2.20
Cereal, wheat flakes	1 cup	2.10
Fig-bar cookies	4 cookies	0.95
Blueberry pie	1 piece	0.94
Cereal, puffed oats	1 cup	0.90
Macaroons	2 cookies	0.80
Spaghetti with tomato sauce and meat	1 cup	0.74
Bran muffins, homemade	1 muffin	0.72
Pumpkin pie	1 piece	0.65
Pecan pie	1 piece	0.59
Apple pie	1 piece	0.54
Peach pie	1 piece	0.54
Mince pie	1 piece	0.54
Bread, wheat, soft—toasted	1 slice	0.50
Roll, hard	1 roll	0.49
Cereal, cornflakes, with sugar	1 cup	0.40
Bread, pumpernickel	1 slice	0.40
Bread, wheat, firm—18 slices/loaf	1 slice	0.40
Bread, wheat, soft—16 slices/loaf	1 slice	0.40
Cereal, cornflakes, plain	1 cup	0.30
Toaster pastries	1 pastry	0.30
Crackers, rye wafers	2 wafers	0.29
Roll, submarine	1 roll	0.27
Banana cream pie	1 piece	0.26
Oatmeal cookies	4 cookies	0.21
Bread, raisin	1 slice	0.20
Devil's food cake, with icing	1 piece	0.20
Macaroni & cheese	1 cup	0.20
Rice, white, long-grain—cooked	1 cup	0.20
Waffles, from mix with eggs & milk	1 waffle	0.20
Pizza, small, with cheese	1 piece	0.18
Pretzel, twisted	10 pretzels	0.18
Rice, white—parboiled	1 cup	0.17
Chocolate chip cookies	4 cookies	0.17
Rice, white, instant	1 cup	0.17
Egg noodles—cooked	1 cup	0.16
Graham crackers	2 crackers	0.15
Popcorn, with oil & salt	1 cup	0.15
Macaroni noodles—cooked	1 cup	0.14

Cherry pie	1 piece	0.14
Brownies	1 brownie	0.14
Spaghetti noodles—cooked	1 cup	0.13
Blueberry muffin	1 muffin	0.12
Pancakes, buckwheat	1 pancake	0.11
Cake, white, with icing	1 piece	0.10
Cake, yellow, with icing	1 piece	0.10
Bagel, egg	1 bagel	0.10
Cupcake, with chocolate icing	1 cupcake	0.10
Bread, rye, light	1 slice	0.10
Cereal, puffed rice	1 cup	0.10
Coffee cake	1 piece	0.10
Biscuit, homemade	1 biscuit	0.10
Bagel, water	1 bagel	0.10
Doughnut, glazed	1 doughnut	0.10
Fruitcake, dark	1 slice	0.10
Bread, white, firm—34 slices/loaf	1 slice	0.10
Bread, white, soft—24 slices/loaf	1 slice	0.10
Bread, white, soft—18 slices/loaf	1 slice	0.10
Cupcake, no icing	1 cupcake	0.10
Sheet cake, no icing	1 piece	0.09
Roll, hamburger	1 roll	0.08
Corn muffin	1 muffin	0.08
Roll, clover	1 roll	0.07
Danish pastry, plain	1 pastry	0.06
Roll, brown & serve	1 roll	0.05
Saltine crackers	4 crackers	0.04
Cookies, sandwich type	4 cookies	0.04
Muffin, plain	1 muffin	0.04
Vanilla wafer cookies	10 cookies	0.04
Pound cake	1 piece	0.03
Gingersnap cookies	4 cookies	0.03
Doughnut, plain	1 doughnut	0.03
Pancakes, plain	1 pancake	0.03
Cereal, puffed corn	1 cup	0.03
Pretzel, stick	10 pretzels	0.01

FOOD	PORTION	GRAMS OF FIBER
Black-eyed peas	½ cup	5.50
Lentils, whole—cooked	1 cup	2.40
Beans, with pork/sweet sauce—canned	½ cup	2.15
Beans, with pork & tomato sauce—canned	½ cup	1.80
Lima beans	½ cup	1.70
Beans, navy, dry—cooked	½ cup	1.40
Sunflower seeds	¼ cup	1.38
Beans, with franks—canned	½ cup	1.30
Beans, red kidney—canned	½ cup	1.15
Brazil nuts, shelled	1 oz	0.90
Peanuts, salted, roasted in oil	¼ cup	0.88
Filberts	¼ cup	0.85
Almonds, chopped	¼ cup	0.85
Coconut, shredded	¼ cup	0.80
Almonds, slivered	¼ cup	0.75
Pecans, chopped	¼ cup	0.68
Walnuts, English	¼ cup	0.63
Pumpkin or squash seeds	¼ cup	0.63
Cashew nuts, roasted in oil	¼ cup	0.50
Peas, split, dry—cooked	½ cup	0.40
Peanut butter	1 tbsp	0.30

LEGUMES, NUTS, AND SEEDS, LISTED BY FIBER CONTENT

SUGARS AND SWEETS, LISTED BY FIBER CONTENT	FOOD	PORTION	GRAMS OF FIBER
	Chocolate, semisweet bits	¼ cup	0.43
	Chocolate-coated peanuts	1 oz	0.30
	Chocolate-flavored syrup, thin	1 oz	0.20
	Jams & preserves	1 tbsp	0.20
	Chocolate-flavored syrup, fudge	1 fl oz	0.20
	Chocolate, plain	1 oz	0.10
	Caramels, plain or chocolate	1 oz	0.10
	Fudge	1 oz	0.10

VEGETABLES AND VEGETABLE PRODUCTS, LISTED BY FIBER CONTENT	FOOD	PORTION	GRAMS OF FIBER
	Bean sprouts, raw	1 cup	4.60
	Broccoli—cooked	1 stalk	2.70
	Brussels sprouts—cooked from raw	1 cup	2.50
	Broccoli, frozen—cooked	1 cup	2.00
	Peas, green—canned	½ cup	1.96
	Brussels sprouts, frozen—cooked	1 cup	1.90
	Beet greens—cooked	1 cup	1.60
	Asparagus tips, frozen—cooked	1 cup	1.60
	Pumpkin—canned	½ cup	1.60
	Corn, sweet, frozen—cooked	1 ear	1.60
	Parsnips—cooked	½ cup	1.55
	Peas, green, frozen—cooked	½ cup	1.52
	Black-eyed peas, frozen—cooked	½ cup	1.30
	Sweet potato—canned	½ cup	1.28
	Cabbage—cooked	1 cup	1.20
	Vegetables, mixed, frozen—cooked	½ cup	1.09
	Sweet potato, boiled, peeled	1 potato	1.06
	Peppers, sweet, raw	1 pepper	1.04
	Peppers, sweet—boiled	1 pepper	1.02
	Asparagus tips—cooked from raw	1 cup	1.00
	Corn, sweet—cooked from raw	1 ear	0.98
	Collards—cooked	½ cup	0.95
	Potato, baked, no skin	1 potato	0.94
	Spinach—canned	½ cup	0.93
	Corn, sweet—canned	½ cup	0.84
	Turnip greens, frozen—cooked	½ cup	0.83
	Sauerkraut—canned	½ cup	0.83
	Spinach, chopped, frozen—cooked	½ cup	0.82
	Beets, whole, cooked, peeled	2 beets	0.80
	Carrot—cooked	½ cup	0.78
	Spinach, leaf, frozen—cooked	½ cup	0.76
	Snap beans, yellow	½ cup	0.75
	Cauliflower, frozen—cooked	½ cup	0.72
	Carrot, raw	1 carrot	0.72
	Lettuce, iceberg	¼ head	0.71
	Snap beans, green	½ cup	0.70
	Beets, cooked, peeled	½ cup	0.70
	Turnips, diced—cooked	½ cup	0.70
	Potato, boiled, no skin	1 potato	0.69
	Tomato, raw	1 tomato	0.68
	Snap beans, wax	½ cup	0.65
	Corn, sweet, cream-style—canned	½ cup	0.64
	Squash, summer—cooked	½ cup	0.63
	Mustard greens—cooked	½ cup	0.63
	Cauliflower—cooked	½ cup	0.63
	Potatoes, hash brown—frozen	½ cup	0.62
	Carrots—canned	½ cup	0.62

Corn, sweet, wet—canned	½ cup	0.58
Cauliflower, raw	½ cup	0.58
Carrot, raw, grated	½ cup	0.55
Spinach—cooked from raw	½ cup	0.54
Okra pods—cooked	5 pods	0.53
Turnip greens—cooked from raw	½ cup	0.51
Asparagus spears, frozen—cooked	4 spears	0.50
Potato salad	½ cup	0.50
French fries—cooked from raw	10 strips	0.50
Tomato juice—canned	1 cup	0.49
Tomato solids—canned	½ cup	0.48
Potatoes, mashed with milk and butter	½ cup	0.42
Corn, sweet, frozen—cooked	½ cup	0.41
Sweet potato—canned	1 piece	0.40
Lettuce, butterhead	¼ head	0.39
Cabbage, raw, shredded	½ cup	0.35
Cabbage, red, raw	½ cup	0.35
Potatoes, mashed—from dehydrated	½ cup	0.32
Potato chips	10 chips	0.32
Onions, young green	6 onions	0.30
Mushrooms, raw	½ cup	0.28
Cabbage, savoy, raw	½ cup	0.28
Onions, raw, chopped	¼ cup	0.26
Celery, raw	1 stalk	0.24
Cabbage, celery, raw	½ cup	0.23
Endive, raw	½ cup	0.23
Celery, raw, diced	¼ cup	0.18
Tomato catsup	1 oz	0.17
Spinach, raw, chopped	½ cup	0.17
Cucumber slices, with peel	6–8 slices	0.17
Radishes, raw	4 radishes	0.13
Cucumber slices, no peel	6–9 slices	0.08
Parsley, raw	1 tbsp	0.06

FOOD	PORTION	GRAMS OF FIBER
Pork/bean soup (canned), with water	1 cup	1.50
Onion soup mix, unprepared	1½ oz	1.04
Minestrone soup (canned), with water	1 cup	0.74
Split pea soup (canned), with water	1 cup	0.64
Tomato vegetable soup, from mix	1 cup	0.50
Cream of tomato soup (canned), with milk	1 cup	0.50
Clam chowder, Manhattan-style (canned), with water	1 cup	0.49
Vegetarian soup (canned), with water	1 cup	0.49
Tomato soup (canned), with water	1 cup	0.49
Cream of mushroom soup, canned, with water	1 cup	0.46
Pickle, cucumber dill	1 pickle	0.33
Vegetable/beef soup, (canned), with water	1 cup	0.32
Cream of mushroom soup (canned), with milk	1 cup	0.25
Onion soup, from mix	1 cup	0.22
Olives, green—canned, with brine	3–4 olives	0.21
Barbecue sauce	1 oz	0.19
Olives, black—canned	2–3 olives	0.14
Cream of chicken soup (canned), with milk	1 cup	0.12
Pickle relish, sweet	1 tbsp	0.12
Cream of chicken soup (canned), with water	1 cup	0.12
Chicken noodle soup, from mix	1 cup	0.07
Mustard, prepared, yellow	1 tsp	0.05

MISCELLANEOUS AND FAST-FOOD ITEMS, LISTED BY FIBER CONTENT

NOTES

INTRODUCTION

1. *The Aerobics Program for Total Well-Being,* Dr. Kenneth H. Cooper (M. Evans and Company, New York, 1982).
2. *Fit or Fat,* Covert Bailey (Houghton Mifflin Company, Boston, 1977). *The Aerobics Program for Total Well-Being,* Cooper.
3. *Fit or Fat,* Bailey.
4. *The Evolution of Human Sexuality,* Donald Symons (Oxford University Press, New York, 1979).

CHAPTER TWO

1. "America's Sweet Tooth," Matt Clark with Mariana Gosnell, Susan Katz, and Mary Hager, *Newsweek,* Aug. 26, 1985, pp. 50–56.
   "Is Salt Really That Bad?," Matt Clark with Deborah Witherspoon, *Newsweek,* Sept. 27, 1982, p. 86.
   "Blood Pressure and Nutrition in Adults: The National Health and Nutrition Examination Survey," *American Journal of Epidemiology,* January 1984, pp. 17–28.
2. *The Pritikin Program for Diet & Exercise,* Nathan Pritikin with Patrick M. Mcgrady, Jr. (Bantam Books, New York, 1983), p. 12.
3. *Fit or Fat,* Covert Bailey (Houghton Mifflin Company, Boston, 1978), p. 88.
4. *Eat to Win,* Dr. Robert Haas (Rawson Associates, New York, 1983), p. 27.
5. *The Pritikin Program for Diet & Exercise,* p. 9.
6. *The Pritikin Program for Diet & Exercise,* p. 11.
7. *The Aerobics Program for Total Well-Being,* Dr. Kenneth H. Cooper (M. Evans and Company, New York, 1982), p. 42.
8. NBC news department.
9. *Fit or Fat,* Bailey, p. 77.
10. *The Pritikin Program for Diet & Exercise,* p. 12.
11. *Fit or Fat,* Bailey, p. 79.
12. *Eat to Win,* Haas, p. 158.
13. *Eat to Win,* Haas, p. 159.
14. *The Pritikin Program for Diet & Exercise,* p. 3.
15. *Fit or Fat,* Bailey, pp. 68–70.
16. *Eat to Win,* Haas, p. 20.
17. *Fit or Fat,* Bailey, pp. 63–76.
18. *Fit or Fat,* Bailey, pp. 81–82.
    Eat to Win, Haas, p. 22.
19. *Eat to Win,* Haas, p. 20.
    Fit or Fat, Bailey, pp. 65–66.
20. *The Pritikin Program for Diet & Exercise,* p. 26.
21. *Fit or Fat,* Bailey, pp. 9–13.
22. *Fit or Fat,* Bailey, pp. 10–13.
23. *Fit or Fat,* Bailey, pp. 3, 71–76.
24. *Fit or Fat,* Bailey, pp. 81–82.
25. *Fit or Fat,* Bailey, pp. 53–58.
26. *Fit or Fat,* Bailey, p. 74.

1. "Effects of Marathon Running, Jogging and Diet on Coronary Risk Factors in Middle-Aged Men," G. H. Hartung, E. J. Farge, and R. E. Mitchell, *Preventative Medicine*, March 1981, pp. 316–323.
   "Sports and Coronary Heart Disease," H. Howald, *Schweiz Med Wochenschr*, Jan. 21, 1984, pp. 110–112.
2. *Fit or Fat*, Covert Bailey (Houghton Mifflin Company, Boston, 1978), p. 19.
   The Aerobics Program for Total Well-Being, Dr. Kenneth H. Cooper (M. Evans and Company, New York, 1982), pp. 107–119.
3. *The Aerobics Program for Total Well-Being*, Cooper, pp. 107–119.
4. *The Aerobics Program for Total Well-Being*, Cooper, p. 124.
5. *The Aerobics Program for Total Well-Being*, Cooper, p. 113.
6. *Fit or Fat*, Bailey, pp. 20–22.
7. *Fit or Fat*, Bailey, pp. 21–28.
   The Aerobics Program for Total Well-Being, Cooper.
8. Lifecycle Company, Bally Fitness Products Corp., 10 Thomas Road, Irvine, California 92714.
9. For preceding exercises:
   Fit or Fat, Bailey.
   The Aerobics Program for Total Well-Being, Cooper.
10. "Jogging the Imagination," A. H. Ismail and L. E. Trachtman, *Psychology Today*, March 1973, pp. 79–82.
11. For preceding aerobic benefits *Fit or Fat*, Bailey.
    The Aerobics Program for Total Well-Being, Cooper.
    The Pritikin Program for Diet & Exercise.

CHAPTER
THREE

1. "Good Health for a Song," Mathew Flamm, *Mademoiselle*, February 1985, pp. 48–49.
2. "Good Health for a Song," Flamm.

CHAPTER
SEVEN

1. *Fit or Fat*, Covert Bailey (Houghton Mifflin Company, Boston, 1978), pp. 50–52.
2. Marc Friedman, M.D., Southern California Sports Medicine Group, Van Nuys, California.
3. Marc Friedman, M.D.
4. Marc Friedman, M.D.
   Prevention & Treatment of Running Injuries, Robert D'Ambrosia, M.D., and David Drez, M.D. (Charles Black, Thoroughfare, New Jersey, 1982).
5. Marc Friedman, M.D.
6. Marc Friedman, M.D.

CHAPTER
EIGHT

CHAPTER NINE

1. "Hot," Susan West, *American Association for the Advancement of Science* magazine, December 1984.
2. "Dietary Carcinogens and Anticarcinogens," Bruce N. Ames, *American Association for the Advancement of Science* magazine, September 1983.
3. *Selenium as Food and Medicine*, Richard A. Passwater, Ph.D. (Keats Publishing, Inc., New Canaan, Connecticut, 1980).
4. "Dietary Carcinogens and Anticarcinogens," Ames.
5. "Cutaneous Malignant Melanoma and Indications of Total Accumulated Exposure to the Sun," C. D. J. Holman and B. K. Armstrong, *National Cancer Institute Journal*, January 1984, pp. 75–82.
   "The Relationship of Malignant Melanoma Basal and Squamous Skin Cancers to Indoor and Outdoor Work," V. Beral and N. Robinson, *British Journal of Cancer*, 1981, pp. 886–891.
6. "A Photobiological Evaluation of Tanning Booths," D. S. Nachtway and R. D. Rundel, *American Association for the Advancement of Science* magazine, 1981.
7. *The Aerobics Program for Total Well-Being*, Dr. Kenneth H. Cooper (M. Evans and Company, New York, 1982).
8. *The Pritikin Program for Diet & Exercise*, Nathan Pritikin with Patrick M. McGrady, Jr. (Bantam Books, New York, 1983).
9. *Life Extension*, Durk Pearson and Sandy Shaw (Warner Books, New York, 1982).
10. Sergeant Bryan Bonessa, California Highway Patrol, in a telephone conversation with the author, January 1985.
11. References for nutrient information:
    Van Nostrand's Scientific Encyclopedia (Van Nostrand Reinhold Company, New York, 1976).
    Life Extension, Pearson and Shaw.
    Holistic Medicine, Kenneth R. Pelletier (Delacorte Press/Seymour Lawrence, New York, 1979).
    The Book of Health, American Health Foundation (Franklin Watts, New York, 1981).
12. *The Book of Health*, American Health Foundation, p. 59.
13. *Life Extension*, Pearson and Shaw, pp. 108–119.
14. *Life Extension*, Pearson and Shaw, pp. 87, 271.
15. *Life Extension*, Pearson and Shaw, p. 411.
16. *Selenium as Food and Medicine*, Passwater, p. 98.